Promoting Nonviolence
in Early Adolescence

Responding in Peaceful and Positive Ways

D1253604

PREVENTION IN PRACTICE LIBRARY

SERIES EDITOR
Thomas P. Gullotta
Child and Family Agency, New London, Connecticut

ADVISORY BOARD

George W. Albee, University of Vermont
Evvie Becker, U.S. Department of Health and Human Services
Martin Bloom, University of Connecticut
Emory Cowen, University of Rochester
Roger Weissberg, University of Illinois
Joseph Zins, University of Cincinnati

BUILDING HEALTHY INDIVIDUALS, FAMILIES, AND COMMUNITIES:
Creating Lasting Connections
Ted N. Strader, David A. Collins, and Tim D. Noe

HIGH-RISK SEXUAL BEHAVIOR:
Interventions with Vulnerable Populations
Evvie Becker, Elizabeth Rankin, and Annette U. Rickel

PROMOTING NONVIOLENCE IN EARLY ADOLESCENCE:
Responding in Peaceful and Positive Ways
Aleta Lynn Meyer, Albert D. Farrell, Wendy Bauers Northup, Eva M. Kung,
and Laura Plybon

REDUCING THE RISKS FOR SUBSTANCE ABUSE:
A Lifespan Approach
Raymond P. Daugherty and Carl Leukefeld

SUCCESSFUL AGING: Strategies for Healthy Living
Waldo C. Klein and Martin Bloom

SUCCESS STORIES AS HARD DATA:
An Introduction to Results Mapping
Barry M. Kibel

TYPE A BEHAVIOR: ITS DIAGNOSIS AND TREATMENT
Meyer Friedman

Promoting Nonviolence
in Early Adolescence

Responding in Peaceful and Positive Ways

Aleta Lynn Meyer
Albert D. Farrell
Virginia Commonwealth University
Richmond, Virginia

Wendy Bauers Northup
Henrico Area Mental Health and Retardation Services
Glen Allen, Virginia

and

Eva M. Kung
Laura Plybon
Virginia Commonwealth University
Richmond, Virginia

Kluwer Academic / Plenum Publishers
New York, Boston, Dordrecht, London, Moscow

Library of Congress Cataloging-in-Publication Data

Promoting nonviolence in early adolescence: responding in peaceful and positive ways/
Aleta Meyer ... [et al.].
   p. cm. — (Prevention in practice library)
   Includes bibliographical references and index.
   ISBN 0-306-46385-7—ISBN 0-306-46386-5 (pbk.)
     1. Conflict management—Study and teaching (Middle school)—United States. 2.
Nonviolence—Study and teaching (Middle school)—United States. 3. Interpersonal
conflict in adolescence—United States—Prevention. I. Meyer, Aleta. II. Series.

HM1126 .P76 2000
303.6'9'071273—dc21

                                        00-029629

ISBN 0-306-46385-7 (Hardbound)
ISBN 0-306-46386-5 (Paperback)

©2000 Kluwer Academic / Plenum Publishers, New York
233 Spring Street, New York, N.Y. 10013

http://www.wkap.nl/

10 9 8 7 6 5 4 3 2 1

A C.I.P. record for this book is available from the Library of Congress

Printed in the United States of America

Preface

In preparation for role-play during a RIPP class, 6th grade students consider the following conflict situation: Sharon and Josie, who are good friends, try out for the basketball team. Josie makes the team, but Sharon does not. The week after tryouts, Sharon tries to pick a fight with Josie, calling her a "cheater" and "someone the coach felt sorry for." Josie is in a bind; she wants to remain friends with Sharon, but she is really angry with Sharon for treating her so badly. What can Josie do in this situation? What type of self-talk will help her work out this problem with Sharon and keep the friendship?

During the role-play, Sharon calls Josie a cheater. Then, before Josie responds, two students representing her positive and negative sides take turns whispering into her ear. Negative self-talk: "Boy, is she a loser! What if everyone believes her and thinks that I cheated to get on the team?!" Positive self-talk: "I know I worked hard to get on the team! Sharon must really be hurt that she didn't make it. I can talk to her later when she's cooled down, and maybe we can do something together after practice." Josie listens to the two voices, and decides that the best approach is to ignore Sharon's comments for now and to call her later that day to see if they can do something together.

This description of students dealing with everyday conflicts is quite real. Although it is the larger tragedies that make the news, these smaller conflicts can build up in a school or a community and lead to more serious problems down the road. As we have witnessed recently across the country, tragic violent events often mobilize a community to demonstrate its concerns. In Detroit, for example, a series of rapes and attempted rapes of young girls on the way to school led to a community where everyone from bus drivers to passing motorists to shop owners pledged to look out for and protect children as they walked to school. In schools where youth themselves have been the cause of the violence, metal detectors have been installed and young people are trained that "telling" on their peers is not betrayal but support for the safety of other students. Many schools are also attempting to help students examine cliques and groups to understand how excluding others can be hurtful.

Although these are important responses to tragic events, we believe that tragedy should not have to occur before a school or community begins making efforts to prevent violence. The fact that violence has never occurred in your school is a perfect reason to begin to take the steps described in this book. RIPP (Responding in Peaceful and Positive Ways) teaches students in middle school how to use techniques and strategies that help them deal with the everyday conflicts. Such seemingly minor conflicts lead teachers to lose valuable teaching time and can, on occasion, escalate into larger tragic events. RIPP also teaches the need for everyone to accept differences, to affirm those with whom they come in contact, and not to engage in "put-downs."

RIPP provides young people with new ways to respond to conflict. The acronym RAID describes four types of nonviolent options: Resolve, Avoid, Ignore, and Diffuse. The program teaches students that they have a choice in any conflict and dispels the notion that "fighting" is a necessary response to an insult or a conflict. It also teaches students a problem-solving model for deciding what to do in a conflict situation. The steps in this model are represented by the acronym SCIDDLE: "Stop, Calm down, Identify the problem and your feelings about it, Decide among your options, Do it, Look back, and Evaluate."

The RIPP program emphasizes a positive approach to conflict through the structure of the lessons and the tone of the classroom. It trains facilitators in active listening and problem-solving skills so that they can model the choices that young people have when faced with a conflict. It develops a level of trust and caring in the classroom so that students can share their experiences and rehearse nonviolent responses to conflict. Finally, the program has been designed with real-life experiences in mind. Young people learn more from their own engagement with activities than they do from information shared with them verbally through lecture.

In this book we describe the program and its history (Chapter 1), how to get RIPP started at a school (Chapter 2), and how to train prevention facilitators to implement RIPP (Chapter 3). We also provide directions on setting up an evaluation plan before the program is implemented (Chapter 4). It is important to know how well the program is working so that adjustments can be made to improve its effectiveness. In Chapters 5 through 7 we describe the curricula and sample workshops to provide a clearer sense of the program's focus and techniques. Finally, we close with a consideration of ways to modify RIPP for specific communities and cultures (Chapter 8).

We hope that you will enjoy reading the book and learning how one violence prevention program worked in several very different communities. More than that, we hope you will be inspired to take the steps necessary to mobilize your school to be proactive about preventing violence to create an environment where young people feel safe and learn the life skills necessary to live in a complex and diverse world.

Acknowledgments

As with any community-based program designed for adolescents, RIPP was developed in collaboration with numerous individuals over many years. We would like to acknowledge these people. Most importantly, we want to thank the violence prevention facilitators who have implemented RIPP and provided us with feedback to improve the program and develop something that can be done in the "real world." Second, we would like to thank the school administrations in our urban and rural settings for their support in program implementation and evaluation. We also extend gratitude and deep appreciation for those who have taken a leadership role regarding violence prevention in these communities: Arthur Johnson, Chris Moore, Sharon Conley, Jack Mosby, and Penny Ginger. We give special thanks to our graduate students who worked on this project early on: Lottie Ampy, Steve Bruce, and Kami White. Warm regards go to Kathy Konrad, Jack Richford, and Micah McCreary for intense conversations regarding the potential of martial arts and adventure activities in violence prevention. We also want to thank Tom Gullotta and Rick Turner, the author/editors who encouraged us to submit a prospectus for this book. Special thanks also go to Lois Farrell for copy editing. We also wish to thank the staff at the Center for Injury and Violence Prevention within the CDC for their commitment to addressing youth violence through the best of research and practice. We are learning!

In closing, the first author would like to extend her deep gratitude to Carole Harder, her high school peer leadership mentor. When Aleta asked Carole why, as an 18-year-old "Senior" peer leader, she was sharing her incredible message and leadership skills with students already identified as leaders, as opposed to every student in the school, she responded quite bluntly, "Aleta, that's *your* job." Thank you, Carole, for that challenge to use the lessons you taught as guidance for effective violence prevention.

Contents

1

Background on Responding in Peaceful and Positive Ways (RIPP):
Violence, Nonviolence, and Positive Risk-Taking in Early Adolescence

OVERVIEW

Although it is the larger tragedies that make the news, smaller conflicts between students can build up in a school or a community and lead to bigger problems. That is why we believe something horrible should not have to occur before a school or community begins to look at ways to prevent violence. The program described in this book was designed to reduce violence and has been effective in both urban and rural settings.

Before a new program is implemented in a school, it is helpful to understand how it evolved. Such information provides insight into the care and attention to detail that went into its development. This is important because the amount of thoughtful effort put into developing a program will inevitably be reflected in the program's overall quality. Because of the care we have taken in developing, evaluating, and refining the Responding In Peaceful and Positive Ways (RIPP) program, we believe it will be useful to those interested in providing a safe, disciplined, and nurturing environment within which to educate their youth.

This chapter provides information about the RIPP program and the methodical process we employed in our efforts to develop a prevention program that would be effective in reducing youth violence. It is our hope that decision-makers will be able to use this information to help guide their own community's efforts to

1

address youth violence. The chapter begins with a description of RIPP and its history. Next, we describe how the program was developed and its goals, objectives, and audience. Then, the findings of several studies that have evaluated the effectiveness of RIPP in two different communities are presented. The chapter concludes with a summary of what we believe works, does not work, and might work.

What is RIPP?

RIPP is the acronym for a violence prevention program for middle and junior high schools titled "Responding In Peaceful and Positive Ways." This program consists of a 25-session curriculum, RIPP-6, designed to be implemented in the 6th grade at middle schools (or 7th grade at junior highs); 12-session booster programs, RIPP-7 and RIPP-8, that are designed to be implemented with 7th and 8th graders at middle schools (or with 8th and 9th graders at junior highs);[1] and a peer mediation program. A prevention facilitator is responsible for teaching the curricula and supervising the peer mediation program. The RIPP curriculum is typically taught in 50-minute sessions on a weekly basis throughout the school year during the academic subjects of social studies, health, and science.

The RIPP program was designed as a primary prevention program for violence to be implemented with the entire student population at a middle or junior high school. The purpose of primary prevention efforts is to reduce the incidence of a particular problem by addressing specific needs within an entire population (Caplan, 1964), as opposed to working with a subgroup of high-risk students within a school. Because of the developmental changes that occur from kindergarten through the middle school years and into high school, youth violence experts argue that there is a need for primary prevention efforts to reduce violence at every stage along that path (Earls, Cairns, & Mercy, 1993). Middle schools and junior highs are particularly important, given that students who attend such schools report lower levels of perceived school safety and higher levels of victimization within the school than those who attend schools with K-8 or K–12 grade configurations (Anderman & Kimweli, 1997).

RIPP employs a valued adult role model to teach students knowledge, attitudes, and skills designed to promote schoolwide norms for nonviolence and positive risk-taking. This is accomplished through the use of team-building activities, a social-cognitive problem-solving model, repetition and mental rehearsal, relaxation techniques, small group work, instruction in specific social skills for preventing violence, role-plays, and a peer mediation program. A key element is a trained prevention facilitator who models prosocial attitudes and behaviors. RIPP-6 is the most extensive of the three curricula and focuses on a wide range of skills

---

[1] For ease of understanding, RIPP-6 will refer to the program taught in the first year, RIPP-7 to the program taught in the second year, and RIPP-8 to the program taught in the third year.

to prevent violence (Meyer & Northup, 1998). RIPP-7 capitalizes on the increasing maturity of the students and focuses on conflict resolution in friendships (Meyer, Northup, & Plybon, 1998). In a similar fashion, RIPP-8 utilizes the natural transition to high school as a tool for encouraging students to apply the skills learned in RIPP to their future lives in high school and adulthood (Meyer & Plybon, 1999).

The peer mediation program provides an ongoing resource that complements the RIPP curricula, as well as the rules and disciplinary procedures in the middle schools. Peer mediators are selected and trained to help students who are having a conflict identify the problem and come to a peaceful resolution. Ideally, the schoolwide peer mediation program provides an opportunity for students to apply the specific skills taught in RIPP to actual conflict situations. Such experiences can add emotional salience to the skills that cannot be provided during a classroom role-play of a conflict (VanSlyck, Stern, & Zak-Place, 1996). In addition, because the successful operation of a mediation program requires coordination throughout the whole school, the peer mediation program helps to establish school norms for addressing conflict in positive ways.

THE HISTORY OF RIPP AND ITS DEVELOPMENT

Background

The history of RIPP began in 1991 when Governor Wilder of Virginia set aside money for school-based violence prevention programs within the state. A Violence Prevention Management Team was created to direct efforts to reduce youth violence in our city. This team was composed of representatives of the city council, the public schools, and the community services board. After deciding to implement a modified version of Prothrow-Stith's (1987) violence prevention curriculum in the middle schools, the team decided it was important to have the effectiveness of the program evaluated. At this point, it recruited one of the authors to conduct a pilot evaluation. This evaluation provided the basis for six years of additional funding through a cooperative agreement with the Centers for Disease Control and Prevention (CDC) which supported evaluations of several promising programs across the United States.

Concerns about the effectiveness of the modified Prothrow-Stith curriculum led us to pursue a different approach. We concluded that there was a strong need for social-cognitive intervention with a clear conceptual framework, clearly stated objectives, and a firm base in research and theory (Farrell, Meyer, & Dahlberg 1996). In 1994 we began developing the RIPP-6 curriculum by developing a conceptual framework and program objectives based on a review of research on relevant topics and a day-long feedback session with the evaluation and implementation teams. During the 1994–1995 school year, prevention facilitators imple-mented a pilot 14-session version of RIPP-6. Our evaluation of this program, review of the curriculum, and feedback from prevention facilitators led to the development of an expanded 25-session curriculum (Meyer & Northup, 1998). This expansion was based on the conclusion that the skills targeted by the inter-vention could not be adequately addressed in 14 sessions and that additional ses-sions were needed to address issues of tolerance and diversity. The resulting 25-session RIPP-6 program is one product of this activity, and the booster programs follow the same iterative path.

The process we used to develop RIPP is often referred to as *action research* (Lewin, 1946). The purpose of action research is to address a social problem through a cyclical process of collaborative problem definition, fact-finding, goal-setting, action, and evaluation that results in an effective program based in both local and research expertise. We believe that our commitment to this process has greatly enhanced our ability to develop a violence prevention program that changes the violent behavior of youth.

Theoretical and Empirical Rationale

The theoretical rationale for RIPP represents an application of Perry and Jessor's (1985) health promotion model for early adolescence. This model is grounded in social-cognitive learning theory, which is based on the assumption that aggression occurs as a function of both individuals and their environments (Bandura, 1989). In particular, a complex set of interactive relationships is thought to exist between people (e.g., developmental factors, cognition, personality vari-ables, motivation, self-efficacy, current physiological state), their behavior, and the environment. Within each of these three domains, there are both health-com-promising factors (i.e., risk factors) and health-promoting factors (i.e., protective factors) (Perry & Jessor, 1985). Consequently, all three domains must be targeted to impact the learning and/or development of violent and nonviolent behavior. This section provides an overview of research and theory on aggressive behavior and early adolescence as it relates to these domains. Implications for developing of effective violence prevention programs (i.e., RIPP) are also discussed. Inter-ested readers are referred to Meyer and Farrell (1998) for a more complete pre-sentation of the rationale for RIPP.

Thoughts and Emotion

A number of theories concerning aggression focus on the thoughts, emo-tions, and physiological states of individuals that can lead to aggressive behavior when something happens to them (i.e., Berkowitz, 1994; Zillman, 1979). In these models, our thoughts affect our emotions and subsequent behaviors. For example, if a person who is shopping at the grocery store is feeling angry about something that happened that day and the grocery clerk does not give the correct change, how that person responds is influenced by the thoughts he or she has at the time. If the person thinks, "Great, another person trying to get one over on me," it is likely that he or she might shout at the clerk. If the person thinks, "Wow, another person besides me doesn't seem to be getting things right today," he or she might politely request that the clerk recount the change. The implications of these theories for prevention are that youths need the following three problem-solving skills. First, they need to learn how to lengthen the reaction time between the triggering event and their response. This extra time creates an opportunity for more complex thoughts to interfere with the aggressive reaction. Second, they need to know how to calm down physiologically in both the short term and the long term. Third, they need to know how to identify their own feelings, clarify the problem, and empathize with others.

Patterns of Thought

Research on cognitive scripts about aggression (e.g., Huesmann & Miller, 1994) and negative attributions (Weiner, Graham, & Chandler, 1982) has focused on thought patterns that set the stage for aggressive responses, regardless of the current emotional or physiological state of a person. Huesmann's (1988) conceptualization of cognitive scripts is based on the idea that much of our behavior and social problem solving is controlled by the things we learned as children that we say over and over in our minds. These thoughts are learned through personal experience or by observing others. A similar idea can be found in research on thoughts called negative attributions (Weiner et al., 1982). This research indicates that people are likely to become angry when they have unpleasant experiences that they attribute to something or someone outside of themselves who they believe could have controlled what happened. Two primary examples of negative attributions concern the way people respond to intentional thwarting (i.e., if they "take the bait") or accidental misdeeds (i.e., if they "expect the worst") (Berkowitz, 1994). Both types of thoughts set the stage for aggressive responses. The implications are that prevention efforts should provide many opportunities for adolescents to (1) critically examine their own thoughts and learn to consider alternative responses, (2) observe nonviolent means of conflict resolution, (3) directly experience the benefits of choosing peaceful options, and (4) practice cognitive scripts for positive behavior.

Social Learning Theory

Patterson and his colleagues have identified three causal processes in the development and continuation of aggressive behavior in youth (Patterson, 1986). The first of these processes occurs as a result of poor family management skills, whereby children learn to use coercive behavior with others (i.e., to use aversive interaction patterns as substitutes for social skills). The second process starts to develop when a child enters school. Children who have learned to be noncompliant and coercive as a way to gain desired outcomes at home are at risk for peer rejection and academic failure in school. In addition, children whose parents cannot manage their behavior are at risk for parental rejection. The implications for prevention in the school setting are to teach faculty and staff to use effective management skills (i.e., monitoring, discipline, positive reinforcement, and involvement). In addition, school-based efforts to prevent violence should provide opportunities to learn friendship skills as well as norms for academic success (Dodge, 1991) because normal peer groups can provide opportunities to learn empathy, reciprocity, cooperation (Bierman, 1989) and because of the value of academic competence (Steinberg, Dornbusch, & Brown, 1992).

Social Information-Processing

Dodge and his colleagues (e.g., Crick & Dodge, 1994; Dodge, 1986) developed a model for understanding children's social adjustment that is based on social information-processing. This model describes children's behavioral responses as a function of their personal capabilities, their memory of past experiences, and the way they process the social cues of any given situation. In other words, how a person responds when faced with a conflict depends on that person's capabilities (e.g., ability to fight, ability to resolve conflicts peacefully), social knowledge (e.g., personal and vicarious memories of the success/failure of various conflict resolution strategies, relationship history), and ability to process social information accurately (e.g., determine the dangerousness of a situation, understand another person's body language). Although the implications of this model for violence prevention are similar to those presented thus far, they warrant being restated using the language of social information-processing. First, the problem-solving model that is taught should be consistent with social information-processing. Second, skills should be taught that enhance the ability of youth to have an accurate understanding of what is happening. Third, the breadth of the social knowledge of youth must be expanded and enriched to include many experiences where they themselves or others experience positive outcomes for choosing to be nonviolent (e.g., opportunities to practice skills in classroom role-plays and peer mediation). The fourth implication is that youth should be provided opportunities to clarify what is important to them (i.e., values) and assess their own behaviors in light of those values.

Situational Factors

Sometimes characteristics of the environment facilitate violent behavior. For example, if a gun is easily accessible in the environment of a person who wants to harm another, it is more likely such harm will occur than if a gun were not available. Friedlander (1993) proposes a model for the way specific situational factors expedite violence when the stage is set by interpersonal risk factors. Given the pervasiveness of situational factors that promote violence (e.g., easy accessibility of weapons, drugs, and alcohol; stereotypes about gender and ethnicity; and advertisements that specialize in encouraging people to "just do it"), it appears that the entire, larger social context of adolescence can set the stage for violence. For this reason, to help youth protect themselves from risky situational factors, efforts to prevent violence and promote desirable alternatives must teach them how to accurately assess the danger of situations before choosing them. Primary prevention efforts should also provide avenues for youth to critically examine the norms and expectations of their schools, communities, and country.

Adolescent Development and Positive Risk-Taking

When considering youth violence, it is important to note that much of the sharp peak in antisocial and violent behaviors that occurs is related to adolescent developmental tasks (Guerra, Tolan, & Hammond, 1994). As youths mature, many new opportunities for conflict arise. For example, peers become the primary focus of relationships, power relationships change in the family, the nature of male–female relationships change, and the need to establish an identity emerges (Crockett & Petersen, 1993). The complexity of the types of social skills and behaviors adolescents must master is reflected in the fact that social competence varies across settings that demand interaction with peers (Bierman & Montminy, 1993). Moreover, skills required in one area (e.g., being agreeable in a close friendship) may conflict with skills required in another area (e.g., resisting peer pressure in a larger social group). This may result in problems if a behavior that is successful in one area (e.g., going along with a friend's idea for solving a problem) is transferred to another area ineffectively (e.g., going along with a large group's decision to experiment with drugs).

The literature on adolescent development has important implications for violence prevention efforts. Increasing adolescents' capacity to respond to developmental challenges in ways that provide opportunities for skill acquisition, personal growth, and the acceptance of personal responsibility is of primary importance. We call this positive risk-taking. One way to accomplish this is to provide structured experiences in a safe, supportive, social environment where youth can practice new behaviors with their peers in small groups. These "risky" experiences should be designed to optimize the chance that youth will understand how similar skills can be applied across multiple settings (i.e., conflict resolution skills can be used now in their present roles as student, friend, and family member and in their future roles as parent, worker, and citizen). Moreover, these structured experiences should capitalize on adolescents' new cognitive abilities by getting them to think critically about the consequences of various courses of action that they or others might take. For example, by reviewing historical figures that overcame tremendous social barriers through nonviolent action (i.e., took positive risks) and helped create life as it is today and by observing the social consequences of those who chose violence, adolescents can learn the connection between action and long-term consequences. In summary, a combination of critical analysis with skill practice can serve the function of increasing resilience while simultaneously decreasing factors that compromise the quality of life.

School Climate

A school climate that values individual students and promotes attitudes and behaviors that respect and protect the rights of others provides a significant protective factor (Remboldt, 1998). Unfortunately, when students are not familiar with other members of their school, there are lower levels of empathy and perspective-taking that decrease the likelihood they will behave prosocially toward each other (Carlo, Fabes, Laible, & Kupanoff, 1999). Moreover, feelings of purposelessness and perceived racism, which includes both objective and subjective experiences, may contribute to the tendency toward a hostile attributional bias (Lochman & Wayland, 1994), which can interfere with accurate social information-processing and lead to aggression (Graham, Hudley, & Williams, 1992). Because of increasing diversity within schools and our society, it is imperative that youth learn to find value in these differences. For this reason, violence prevention efforts in schools must employ ground rules that value the dignity of each person (e.g., We will listen to each other, "Put-downs" are not allowed). In addition, such efforts should engage students in interactive processes that help them learn more about each other as people. These processes can range from simple team-building games to thoughtfully facilitated discussions about gender, ethnicity, heritage, and culture. Finally, efforts to promote a positive school climate in middle and junior high schools will be most effective if initiated at the beginning of the transitional year (e.g., the 6th grade for middle schools) and extended throughout the entire school year.

Nonviolence

It is important to describe the word "nonviolence" as a process that is much more than the absence of violence. Nonviolence involves the active cultivation of agreements and often requires more energy and time than violence (Cox, 1986). A core foundation for nonviolence is the belief that there are connections among all people and that it is therefore possible for both parties in a conflict to "win" (Crum, 1987). This implies the need for activities that promote mutual respect and that push individuals to focus on the goal of attaining the best outcome for all involved.

Lessons Learned from Violence Prevention Programs

In addition to incorporating our own lessons learned in violence prevention, we have worked diligently to incorporate state-of-the-art knowledge about other effective and promising programs into our school-based efforts (e.g., Dusenbury, Falco, Lake, Brannigan, & Bosworth, 1997; Howard, Flora, & Griffin, 1999; Samples & Aber, 1998) . For example, our conclusions about the value of interactive techniques for skill-building are affirmed by Dusenbury et al.'s (1997) report summarizing the critical elements of promising violence prevention programs. In this report, the authors also highlighted the need for programs to be developmentally appropriate, to be focused on skill-building (e.g., anger management, perspective-taking, problem-solving, listening), to be matched to the ethnic identity and culture of the students, to provide extensive staff development and teacher training for program implementers, and to promote a positive school climate with norms against violence and aggression. In addition to outlining strategies that are most promising, their report highlighted components of programs that may not work or that have negative effects. Their conclusions are consistent with the lessons we have learned through our own efforts to develop an effective violence prevention program. For example, using scare tactics, such as graphic pictures of videos of violent scenes, is more likely to promote violent behavior than to deter it. The same is true for strategies that segregate aggressive or antisocial students. Finally, these reviewers argued that, whereas implementing programs in schools that are already overwhelmed may serve to weaken the system rather than strengthen it, programs that are too brief or focused only on information or self-esteem may lead to many unfulfilled expectations.

Program Objectives for RIPP

In the process of identifying specific objectives for RIPP, we attempted to develop a rationale that was both sensible to those implementing the program and consistent with developmental theory and research. Each of the 12 objectives we identified falls under one of the three domains specified by social learning theory (Bandura, 1989): intrapersonal factors, behavioral factors, and environmental factors, and is directly related to important developmental tasks for early adolescents. These objectives are also consistent with Perry and Jessor's (1985) model for transforming developmental theory into objectives for health-promotion programs because they include health-promoting factors that need to be increased and health-compromising factors that need to be reduced. In summary, the goal of RIPP is to implement strategies that reduce risk factors (i.e., health-compromising factors) and increase protective factors (i.e., health-promoting factors), which will then lead to less violent behavior and more positive behavior.

A. Environmental Objectives (expectations and opportunities in the environment)
   1. Develop norms and expectations for nonviolent means of conflict resolution and positive achievement.
   2. Create opportunities for conflict resolution and positive achievement.
   3. Provide adult and peer models for conflict resolution and positive achievement.
   4. Provide institutional and peer support for conflict resolution and positive achievement.
B. Intrapersonal Objectives (knowledge, attitudes, and beliefs inside the individual)
   5. Provide knowledge to support the value of nonviolent conflict resolution and positive achievement.
   6. Develop values that sustain nonviolent conflict resolution and positive achievement.
   7. Diminish stereotypes, beliefs, attributions, and cognitive scripts that support violence.
   8. Develop cognitive scripts for prosocial behavior.
C. Behavioral Objectives (skills and abilities of the individual)
   9. Enlarge skills repertoire for nonviolent conflict resolution and positive achievement.
   10. Provide experience in mentally rehearsing nonviolent means of conflict resolution and positive achievement.
   11. Promote self-management through repeated use of problem-solving models.
   12. Enlarge ability of participants to identify the optimal violence prevention strategy in a given situation and given personal skills and values.

These 12 objectives provide the groundwork for the RIPP program. For example, the ground rules that are established for RIPP-6 create a norm of respecting others. A classroom environment and valued adult role model that maintain this norm facilitate the likelihood that students will take positive risks, such as participating in a role-play in front of the group. Such role-plays allow for the practice of new skills. For students who have never tried talking through a conflict with another, role-playing can foster a positive attitude about the utility of this approach to resolving conflicts. For students watching role-plays, observing positive conflict resolution can serve to reinforce positive social norms, as well as provide an opportunity to mentally rehearse prosocial behavior.

WHO IS RIPP FOR?

The RIPP program was originally developed to meet the needs of public school students in a mid-sized city in the southeastern United States. Like most urban areas, violence is a serious problem in this community. Students from these public schools are largely from minority and economically disadvantaged families who live in neighborhoods where crime and drug use are high. Nearly 90% are African-American and the majority (60%) live in single-parent, female-headed households (Farrell et al., 1992). Data from a sample of 496 sixth graders collected at the beginning of the 1994 school year reflect the frequency with which these students are exposed to violence in their communities (Farrell, Meyer, & Dahlberg, 1996). More than 92% reported hearing gunshots in their neighborhood, more than 78% reported having seen someone arrested, more than 84% reported having seen someone beaten up, and 43% of the boys and 31% of the girls reported having seen someone get shot. These youth are not just witnesses but also frequently victims and perpetrators. According to their own reports, among boys, 70% had been in a physical fight, 8% had been injured in a fight, 10% had been threatened by someone with a weapon, and 16% had threatened someone with a weapon during the previous 30 days. Among girls, 44% had been in a physical fight, 5% had been injured in a fight, 2% had been threatened by someone with a weapon, and 5% had threatened someone with a weapon in the previous 30 days. In many cases, these youth feel pressure to fight; 46% of the boys and 36% of the girls reported feeling pressure from their friends to fight someone during the past 30 days.

Although designed for an urban school system, RIPP has more recently been implemented in a rural school system in the southern United States. This opportunity arose when a group of four rural school districts received funding from the United States Department of Education to replicate RIPP (Valois, Tidwell, & Farrell, 1999). The student population in this rural system differs from our original urban population because it is rural and also because of the diversity of the students. An overall snapshot of this project would depict a student population that was 45% Caucasian, 24% Hispanic, 13% African-American, and 18% who described themselves as "Other." The "Other" category in itself is a unique melting pot of ethnicity, whereby students report multiple combinations of parental ethnicity. Baseline data from the pilot evaluation of the project in the rural area clearly indicate that violence among students is not restricted to urban communities. For example, in the past 30 days, 40% of students reported that they had been in a physical fight, 6% that they had brought a weapon to school, 8% that they had been injured in a fight and required medical treatment, and 33% that they felt pressured by their friends to fight someone. In terms of lifetime exposure to community violence, 51% reported that they had seen someone they did not know get beat up, 14% reported having seen a stranger get shot, and 10% reported having seen a stranger killed (Valois et al., 1999).

Whereas RIPP was created to meet the needs of students in what were considered high-risk communities, the empirical research and developmental theory on which RIPP is based (e.g., Crockett & Petersen, 1993; Dodge, 1986; Garbarino, 1982; Huesmann, 1988; Patterson, 1986) reflects a wider range of communities throughout the United States. In spite of the tremendous variability in culture across and within school communities in our country, all schools share a common commitment—to provide a safe, disciplined, and nurturing environment within which to educate students and socialize them for the adult roles of citizen, family member, and worker. For this reason, we expect that RIPP will be an appropriate violence prevention program for many middle and junior high schools, not just those identified at high-risk, as more and more schools become aware of their own desire to purposefully promote schoolwide norms for nonviolent behavior.

HOW EFFECTIVE IS RIPP?

In this section we summarize the findings of outcome studies we have conducted to examine the effectiveness of RIPP. As noted previously, the RIPP curricula represent the end products of a series of studies in which we implemented a version of each program, evaluated its impact, and then revised it based on our evaluative findings. This section does not describe all this developmental work but instead focuses on our evaluations of the current versions of these programs. These include studies that examined the impact of RIPP-6 and RIPP-7 in two different communities (Farrell, Meyer, Sullivan, & Kung, in preparation; Farrell, Meyer, & White, 1999; Valois et al., 1999). In this section, we give an overview of the findings of these studies. Readers interested in additional details regarding the methodology and findings of these studies should refer to the original reports.

Impact of RIPP-6 in an Urban Public School System

Our evaluation of the 25-session RIPP-6 curriculum began during the 1995–1996 school year. We evaluated the impact of RIPP-6 at three middle schools in an urban public school system using a within-school design. Classrooms of 6th graders in each school were randomly assigned to participate in RIPP-6 or to a no-intervention comparison group (Farrell, Meyer, & White, 1999). Students in special education classrooms were not included in this study. Students completed a battery of outcome measures assessing attitudes, knowledge, and behaviors that we expected to be influenced by the intervention at the beginning and end of the 1995–1996 and 1996–1997 school years. This provided data to compare the groups before and after the intervention and at 6-month and 12-month follow-up. We were also able to collect data on disciplinary code violations and suspensions from each school.

A total of 626 students participated in this evaluation; 305 students participated in RIPP-6, and 321 were in the control group. Both groups were about evenly divided between boys and girls. As previously noted in this chapter, this school system serves a predominantly African-American student population, many of whom come from low-income families. Those assigned to the intervention attended an average of 21 of the 24 sessions; 16 students missed half or more of the sessions. Baseline and post-test data on school disciplinary code violations were available for nearly all participants (98%). Self-report measures were missing due to absentees, students who elected not to complete the measures, and students who provided measures with apparent patterns of random responding. Transfers to different schools resulted in the loss of disciplinary data on 143 of the 626 students at the follow-up assessments.

Analyses were completed on an intention-to-treat basis in which all participants assigned to RIPP were included in the intervention group, regardless of their attendance. These analyses examined intervention effects after accounting for any differences that may have been due to gender or school differences. We also compared the effects of the intervention on boys and girls to determine if there were any differential gender differences. Finally, a random sample of each prevention facilitator's classes was observed to make sure that the program was implemented properly.

Significant program effects were found on several important outcome variables at post-test. Compared to students in the control group, students who participated in RIPP-6

- were less likely to have disciplinary code violations for carrying weapons (0.9% vs. 3.8%),
- were less likely to have in-school suspensions (0.9% vs. 4.4%),
- had lower reported rates of fight-related injuries (2.7% vs. 6.4%),
- were more likely to participate in their school's peer-mediation program (41.5% vs. 29.5%), and
- received higher scores on a test assessing knowledge of the material covered in the curriculum (9.3 vs. 7.4 correct answers).

At the 6-month follow-up, effects were maintained on in-school suspensions, participation in peer mediation, and mastery of the intervention material. Although post-test treatment effects for disciplinary code violations for carrying weapons and reports of fight-related injuries were not maintained at follow-up, this was partially due to attrition (i.e., many students caught carrying weapons in the 6th grade were no longer at school in the 7th grade). Two new intervention effects emerged at the 6-month follow-up. Compared to the comparison group, participants in RIPP-6 were less likely to report that they had threatened to hurt or harm a teacher (14.5% vs. 23.8%). The second effect was specific to boys. Boys who participated in RIPP-6 were less likely than boys who did not to report that they skipped school because they were concerned about their safety (3.8 vs. 12.1%). Two significant differences were still apparent at the 1-year follow-up. Participants in RIPP-6 continued to score higher on the test assessing their mastery of the curriculum and were more likely to report that they had participated in peer mediation.

Although the results of this evaluation were generally encouraging, intervention effects were not found for all of the self-report measures of attitudes and behaviors targeted by the intervention. The maintenance of several effects at the 6-month follow-up was an important finding in that it indicated that the effects of the program could be sustained into the next school year. The fact that these effects were not maintained at the 1-year follow-up underscores the need for RIPP-7 which is designed to sustain and build upon the effects of RIPP-6.

Impact of RIPP-6 in a Rural Public School System

In 1997, we began collaborating on a replication of the RIPP program in a rural area with a consortium of four school districts (Valois et al., 1999). During the 1997–1998 school year, the RIPP-6 program was implemented at five of these schools, and four other schools within the same counties served as control schools. This sample was more diverse in terms of ethnicity than the urban sample; 56% were described as White or Caucasian, 26% as Hispanic or Latino; and 14% as African-American or Black. Although the RIPP-6 program is designed to be implemented across the full school year, the starting date for this project prevented that from happening during the pilot year. The prevention facilitators completed training during January 1997 and implemented the program during the second semester of the school year. One consequence of this schedule was that it was not possible to implement the RIPP-6 program with all the students at each of the intervention schools. Two schools in particular had low rates of participation in RIPP-6 (i.e., 20% and 42%). Rates of participation at the other three intervention schools ranged from 81% to 96%. A second consequence of the delayed starting date was that prevention facilitators had to be creative in developing implementation plans to serve as many students at their schools as possible over a short period of time. For example, sessions at one school were held daily rather than weekly. This pilot implementation did provide an opportunity to examine the impact of RIPP-6 using two different designs—one involving a comparison between several schools and the other a comparison of students within one of the schools. Results of these evaluations need to be interpreted cautiously, however, because of the various modifications needed to implement RIPP-6 within a single semester of the school year.

The between-school evaluation of RIPP-6 included the three schools that had fairly high rates of implementing RIPP-6 and the four control schools where RIPP was not implemented with any students. Data on a battery of outcome measures were obtained at the beginning and end of the school year from 379 (57%) students at the three intervention schools and 532 (48%) of the students at the four control schools. Analyses were completed on an intention-to-treat basis; all students at the intervention schools were included in the intervention group whether they actually participated in the program or not (see Valois, Tidwell, & Farrell, 1999 for a more detailed report of these findings). Although this is a fairly conservative approach, it provides a more realistic evaluation of the impact of attempting to implement a program schoolwide. These analyses examined intervention effects after accounting for any differences that may have been due to gender or ethnicity. We also examined differences in the impact of the program across gender and ethnicity.

As expected, students at the three intervention schools obtained significantly higher scores on an intervention knowledge test than students at the control schools. Although significant program effects were not found on summary measures of problem behaviors and attitudes, significant effects were found for several specific behaviors at the end of the school year. Compared to students at the intervention schools, those at control schools were more likely to report that they had skipped school in the past 30 days because they were worried about their safety. Students at control schools were also more likely to report that they had carried a weapon, been injured in a fight such that they required medical treatment, and used a variety of drugs (i.e., cigarettes, beer, wine, liquor, marijuana, inhalants, and cocaine).

A within-school evaluation of RIPP-6 was conducted at the school where only half the students had participated in RIPP-6. Students at this school were assigned to the intervention or control group based on "pods." Students are assigned to "pods" (sometimes referred to as teams at other schools) at the beginning of the school year. According to the principal, this assignment is essentially random. One pod, which consisted of 102 students, was assigned to the RIPP program and the other pod, which consisted of 144 students, served as a control group. Complete pretest and post-test data were available from 170 students (69%), including 76 students in the intervention group and 94 in the no-treatment control group.

Comparisons of pre- and postintervention data revealed significant differences on several outcome measures between students who participated in RIPP-6 and those who did not:

- A pre-to-post increase in the frequency of drug use was reported by students who did not participate in the program, but not by those who participated.

- Nonparticipants reported greater increases in their frequency of physical violence (i.e., a composite measure of behaviors such as physical fighting and threatening other students and teachers).
- Nonparticipants showed greater increases in attitudes favoring the use of violence.
- Among boys, nonparticipants reported greater pre-to-post increases in nonphysical aggression (e.g., insults and spreading rumors).
- Among girls, nonparticipants reported greater pre-to-post increases in peer provocation.
- Students who participated in RIPP got significantly more items correct on a test assessing mastery of the curriculum than those who did not (i.e., 8.3 versus 6.1).
- Nonparticipants were 3.6 times more likely to report having threatened to hurt or physically harm another student, 3.6 times more likely to report having shoved or pushed another student, 1.9 times more likely to report they had hit or slapped another kid, 2.7 times more likely to report that they had been drunk, 3.0 times more likely to report beer use, 3.1 times more likely to report wine use, and 3.8 times more likely to report liquor use (all based on the past 30 days).

Impact of RIPP-7 in an Urban Public School System

Our evaluation of the 12-session RIPP-7 curriculum began during the 1997–1998 school year. We evaluated the impact of RIPP-7 at two middle schools in the urban school system using a within-school design. Classrooms of 7th graders at each school were randomly assigned to participate in RIPP-7 or to a no-intervention comparison group (Farrell, Meyer, Sullivan, & Kung, in preparation). Students completed a battery of outcome measures assessing attitudes, knowledge, and behaviors that we expected to be influenced by the intervention at the beginning and end of the 1997–1998 and 1998–1999 school years. We were also able to collect data on disciplinary code violations and suspensions from each school. At this point, we have completed analyses of program effects through the 6-month follow-up.

A total of 466 students participated in the evaluation; 219 students participated in RIPP-7, and 247 students were in the control group. Both groups were about evenly divided between boys and girls; the majority of students (96%) were African-American. Pre- and post-test data were available for 163 students in the intervention group and 186 in the control group. Analyses were conducted to examine intervention effects after controlling for the influence of gender and school effects.

Significant program effects were found on several important outcome variables at post-test. Compared to the control group, RIPP-7 participants showed a significant increase in their knowledge of the curriculum material and a trend for greater decreases in anxiety. Significant differences in the impact of the program on boys and girls were found for reported use of wine and in-school suspensions. Boys who did not participate in RIPP-7 were 2.1 times more likely to report using wine in the past 30 days than students who participated in the intervention. A similar effect was not found for the girls. Although the prevalence of in-school suspensions was lower among boys who participated in RIPP-7 compared to those who did not, the opposite effect was found for girls (i.e., participants were more likely to have in-school suspensions).

Effects on knowledge of the curriculum material and anxiety were maintained at the 6-month follow-up, and several additional intervention effects emerged. Compared to students in the no-intervention control group, students who participated in RIPP-7 showed a significant increase in prosocial responses to hypothetical problem situations. Among boys, RIPP participants reported a slight decrease in drug use, in contrast to boys in the control group who reported an increase. Students in the control group were 2.3 times more likely to report bringing a weapon to school than students in the intervention group. Students in the control group were 2.1 times more likely to report wine use than students in the intervention group. Among boys, those in the control group were 3.8 times more likely to have had a disciplinary code violation for violent behavior (i.e., fighting, assault, weapons) than boys in the intervention group.

Impact of RIPP-7 in a Rural Public School System

Our collaboration on the replication of RIPP in a rural setting also provided an opportunity to evaluate RIPP-7. RIPP-7 was implemented during the 1997–1998 school year at the same five middle schools where RIPP-6 had been implemented the previous year. Data on student reports were obtained from students at these intervention schools and from students at the four control schools. We were also able to obtain data on school disciplinary code violations for seven of these schools. The percentage of students who participated in RIPP-7 varied from 60% to 92% across schools, and an average of 74% of students participated. Although RIPP-7 was designed to be implemented with students who had already participated in RIPP-6, not all students at the intervention schools had participated in RIPP-6 during the previous school year. The percentage of students at the intervention schools who participated in both RIPP-6 and RIPP-7 ranged from 11% to 60%, averaging 37% across schools.

A between-school analysis was conducted on data obtained from students at four of the intervention schools and three of the control schools. One intervention school and one control school were not included in this evaluation because data were collected from a fairly low percentage of students at these schools. The impact of RIPP-7 was evaluated by comparing data collected at the end of the 7th grade to pretest data that had been collected at the beginning of the 6th grade. Because many students at the intervention schools had also participated in RIPP-6 during the time between the two data collection points, it is not possible to determine the extent to which any observed changes were uniquely related to RIPP-7 versus the combined effect of both programs. Pre-and-post data were obtained from a total of 448 (39%) of the students at the four intervention schools and 272 (40%) of the students at the three control schools. Analyses were again conducted on an intention-to-treat basis, and differences due to gender, ethnicity and differences across schools were controlled for before examining program effects (see Valois et al., 1999 for a more detailed report of these findings).

Significant program effects were found on several important outcome variables at post-test. Compared to the control group, RIPP-7 participants obtained significantly higher scores on the test assessing their knowledge of the intervention material. They also reported lower rates of peer pressure to use drugs. Although significant program effects were not found on other summary measures of problem behaviors and attitudes, significant intervention effects were found for several specific behaviors. Compared to students at the intervention schools, those at control schools were more likely to report that they had threatened to hit or harm another child, had hit or slapped another child, and had been threatened or injured by someone with a weapon in the past 30 days. Students at control schools were also more likely to report that they had carried a weapon, been in trouble with the police or court system, used liquor, and smoked marijuana.

Analyses were also conducted to compare prevalence rates of disciplinary referrals and violations using data obtained from four of the intervention schools and three of the control schools. These analyses indicated that, compared to students at the intervention schools, students at the control schools were 1.8 times more likely to have had disciplinary referrals and were 1.9 times more likely to have had disciplinary violations related to violent incidents (e.g., fighting, assault, bringing weapons to school). These changes were based on the spring semester after controlling for any differences at the end of the previous school year.

Conclusions

The findings of several evaluation studies provide encouraging support for the effectiveness of the RIPP intervention. Results of the evaluation of RIPP-6 in an urban setting found positive effects at post-test and at a 6-month follow-up. Results of an evaluation of a pilot implementation at a school in the rural system suggest that the program may be effective in the school system where it was developed and also in other settings that serve a very different student population. Of particular note in this study were the significant effects on reported rates of drug use. Analyses of the impact of RIPP-7 in both settings suggest that participants in this program are less likely to show the increase in violent behaviors and other problem behaviors, such as drug use, evident among students who do not participate in the program.

Although we are encouraged by these findings, considerable work remains to be done. We are currently completing an evaluation of RIPP-8. The results of this evaluation will indicate whether this curriculum is effective in its present form or whether additional revisions are needed. The effectiveness of RIPP in school systems that differ from the urban setting in which it was developed also remains to be seen. The results of the pilot evaluation in a rural setting were encouraging and we are looking forward to completing a larger scale evaluation of the full 3-year program in a nine-school between-school design. Thus, the evaluative studies described in this section represent more of a starting point than an end point. Although the program appears promising, it will be important to continue to evaluate its effectiveness as it is implemented in new settings. This topic will be examined further in Chapter 4 where we describe methods for evaluating new implementations of RIPP.

SUMMARY

What Works:

- Hiring a qualified full-time prevention facilitator to implement RIPP.
- Implementing the 25-session RIPP-6 curriculum once a week for a year the first year of middle school or junior high.
- Combining the RIPP curriculum with a schoolwide peer mediation program.
- Using developmentally appropriate activities.
- Basing a program in social learning theory, with a focus on skills, attitudes, and the social environment.
- Starting the program at the beginning of a transitional year (i.e., 6th grade in middle school; 7th grade in junior high).

What Doesn't Work:

- Using informational strategies alone.
- Implementing a brief program.
- Utilizing inadequately trained teachers.
- Using scare tactics.
- Implementing an intensive program in an already overloaded school.

What Might Work:

- Using adequately trained academic teachers or health instructors to implement RIPP.
- Implementing RIPP-6 alone.
- Implementing RIPP-7 alone.

2

Getting RIPP Running

The task of setting up a violence prevention program may seem a little overwhelming. This may be especially true for schools that are about average in student disruptions and where staff may not perceive that there is much of a problem. Unfortunately, in many such schools the number of student conflicts may be growing and many disagreements may be close to escalating into fights. There are thus good reasons for being proactive and establishing a program such as RIPP within a school before serious problems develop. This chapter was designed to assist in that process. Based on our experiences with RIPP, we have identified six conditions that appear particularly important in making the program effective. Specifically, these conditions are (1) a schoolwide commitment to preventing violence; (2) a core group of school staff who serve as advocates for RIPP; (3) a qualified, full-time violence prevention facilitator; (4) adequate training for the violence prevention facilitator in RIPP and peer mediation; (5) willingness by the school staff to incorporate the RIPP and peer mediation programs throughout the school year; and (6) establishing and evaluating objectives for implementing RIPP.

This chapter provides guidelines for promoting these conditions, as well as suggestions for improvising if it is not possible to establish these conditions within a school. This chapter was written to provide the type of practical information that is needed by someone interested in implementing RIPP within a school. To facilitate such efforts, we have written this chapter much like a dialogue we would have with such a person. More specifically, we describe

- ways to determine a school's (or district's) readiness to get started,
- ideas for gaining a schoolwide commitment to preventing violence,
- ways to figure out how much RIPP will cost and how to pay for it,
- criteria for hiring a RIPP facilitator,

- methods for incorporating RIPP and a peer mediation program into a school,
- obstacles that might be encountered along the way, and
- suggestions for modifying the implementation of RIPP if funds for hiring a full-time facilitator are not available.

SCHOOL READINESS

Before starting something new at a school, it is extremely important to assess the school's level of readiness. If teachers and administrators believe that an increasing amount of their time is taken up with student discipline, leaving them little time to teach class material, they may be ready to hear about RIPP. Not all student violations appear to be related to interpersonal conflict and the disciplinary code may be adequate to deal with such infractions. Many violations are, however, related to interpersonal conflict. For example, school codes such as fighting and class disruption are directly related to student interpersonal conflicts. Many disciplinary systems do not attempt to solve the interpersonal component of these problems, and students return from detentions or suspensions with the initial conflict still festering. This sets the stage for continued discipline problems.

Although the link between interpersonal conflict and school disruption may be clear to some, not everyone may see the same link. Members of a school faculty that sense a need for a violence prevention program at their school may wish to gather data to make this case. One possibility is to collect data on school suspensions and their causes and to use these data to demonstrate how the frequency of school suspensions is hindering the school's ability to achieve its mission. It may be helpful to conduct a poll of teachers or hold focus groups to determine the amount of class time spent dealing with interpersonal disputes between students. Another useful strategy may involve enlisting the aid of key people in the system. If you are not an administrator, you might get a principal or assistant principal on your side. If you are an administrator, try building support among influential teachers. Tap into the school's informal network of social communication as a way to build support.

If your role is outside of the school boundaries, such as membership in a local youth agency or parent advocacy group, many of the previously mentioned strategies for gathering support will be useful to you as well. Unfortunately, many programs that come from the outside fade out over time because of lethargy—you may not be able to reach the people you need or teachers may keep forgetting that this program is coming into their classroom. This is why it is so important to build pockets of support within the administration and the teachers and staff; the more closely related you are to the school community, the better your chances of success. For example, an influential retired teacher or administrator who is convinced of the need for RIPP and is willing to work with you as an advocate can get appointments and find inroads that you may not be able to locate.

SCHOOL COMMITMENT

Once there is agreement to establish the program in the school or district, you will need to begin developing an infrastructure to ensure an ongoing commitment. Because the overall goal of the program needs to be clear to everyone, reviewing the school's mission and how promoting positive ways of interacting serves that mission is an important first step. Next, the specific objectives of the program need to be identified. For example, when we first began to put violence prevention into the system with which we were working—a medium-sized urban school system—we received such comments as "I thought you were going to end violence; what are you actually doing about it?" Others thought they should see a quick and dramatic decline in violent youth crimes in the city. In other words, because the program was called a "violence prevention" program, it was assumed that the program purported to directly address the level of violence occurring in the larger community. In fact, the goal of RIPP is to promote nonviolence in the school setting by teaching youth more effective ways of dealing with interpersonal conflicts than fighting and by lowering the number of violent incidents in the school setting. Reducing violent crime among youth is a noble goal. If schools are successful in implementing violence prevention programs in comprehensive ways, that goal may eventually be reached. But that is not the immediate goal of RIPP or any similar program that you may be considering. Meeting with the administration and staff to decide exactly what they want to accomplish with this program and helping them put it into simply understood and energizing terms is a very worthwhile enterprise.

A simple way to initiate the development of school-level goals and short-term objectives for the program is to meet with the staff and get them to brainstorm about the things that they would like to see change—or would like to prevent—in the school as a result of the RIPP program. Divide them into small groups, and ask then to write down three or four things that each would like to see as a result of the program. Ask the groups to discuss the various ideas generated and select the three or four most important. It is likely that many people will have said the same things in different words and much of this exercise will be choosing the wording they all can agree on. Next, have them write their four top priorities on separate notes. Have individuals call out the priorities they have come up with as you go around the room and pin each note to a sheet of poster board.

After all of the ideas have been randomly placed on the poster board (each one having been spoken aloud as it was being put up), ask the staff to get up, walk to the poster, and group the ideas as they see fit. Everyone should be up and milling around the poster board at the front of the room. You will find that they will begin discussing the various suggestions and how they should be grouped. People will flow to the front and then drop back after a few minutes of activity. At the end, there will be almost no switching left, and most of the notes will be grouped together. Now ask the teachers to give each of those groupings a title: e.g., Less Fighting; Conflict Resolution Skills; Better Academic Performance; etc. If you immediately notice some idea that is clearly beyond the scope of the program, such as reducing the availability of firearms in the community, you might get the teachers to discuss the possibility of achieving that with a school-based program.

After this meeting, you can draft a goal statement incorporating the ideas which the staff felt were the most important outcomes of the program. At a later meeting, you can bring the draft back, and the staff can react to it and suggest changes they may now deem pertinent.

Once you have written the goal statement, it is important to define a clear set of measurable objectives for what you want to accomplish. These should include both short-term (1-year) and long-term (3-year) time frames, so that expectations for immediate results do not get built up. It is important to remember that the problems with youth violence did not happen overnight and the most comprehensive program will not change them quickly. Some appropriate objectives might be to decrease the number of detentions or suspensions in the school, improve school climate, decrease the time teachers or administrators spend on disciplinary matters, improve students' communication and conflict resolution skills, or improve relationships among culturally or ethnically diverse groups.

ESTABLISHING A CORE GROUP OF SUPPORT

The final task in preparing to implement the program is creating a management team to oversee the various aspects of the program. Because this team will endure over time, it will fulfill different roles at different times. Its exact composition will depend on whether the program is schoolwide or systemwide. Within a single school, you would want a principal, a guidance counselor, the school security guard or resource office from the local police, perhaps the in-school suspension supervisor or the risk- or drop-out-prevention specialist (if there is one), along with the RIPP facilitator. If the program is systemwide, you might consider the same classifications of people at the system level. If the implementation of RIPP is a cooperative arrangement with a nonschool agency, the director of that office should also serve on the management team.

The members of the management team have a variety of responsibilities. They should be problem-solvers and barrier-busters. They are the group who, sitting in the room together, can make things happen that can ensure the smooth implementation of the program. If additional funds are needed for an assembly or some other project, these are the people who can come forward with those funds. If the facilitator is experiencing resistance from teachers, this is the group that can find a solution.

This is also the group that will decide how to promote the program. For example, all teachers will have to become aware of the program, and steps will need to be taken to ensure that as many "buy into it" as possible. In our experience, the more the whole school begins to be changed by the RIPP program, the more effective the program is in making the necessary changes in school climate. The management team will need to spend some time strategizing on the best ways to bring everyone on board.

Finally, the management team is the support network vital to making the program a success. So the wider its tentacles, the more effective it will be. School violence and conflict affect a wide range of concerns in a school or a system. The management team needs to be deeply committed to the success of the program and make whatever efforts are necessary to ensure that success. One component of this success may be for the management team to ask itself, "What would a school look like that has a commitment to promoting nonviolence, not just preventing violence?"

COSTS OF THE PROGRAM

The original RIPP program and replications of RIPP that have been effective have all followed a model in which a full-time violence prevention facilitator was hired and trained for each school. Although this may appear to be expensive, we have experimented with models where personnel were split across two or more schools or where members of the academic teaching staff were trained to implement the program. In each case, our experience indicates that such models diminish the impact of the RIPP program. Because we believe that an investment in the prevention of violence will greatly offset the future cost of "unprevented" youth violence, this section describes the costs of the RIPP program assuming that one violence prevention facilitator per school will be hired. Suggestions for modifying RIPP if such an arrangement is not possible are provided at the end of the chapter.

The primary cost of the program is the facilitators' salary. Because qualified applicants for this position must have a bachelor's degree in human services or a related field and experience in working with children, the salary for this position should be similar to that of teaching staff with similar levels of education and experience. Determining when to bring staff on-line is one component of this decision. Clearly, the best time to begin a program is at the beginning of the school year. Hiring staff members at least a month earlier assures that they have adequate training and gives them time to get to know the school and the schedule on which they will be working. Then, they can have some sense of confidence when they begin working with teachers after school starts.

Secondary costs for the program include training and materials. An intensive training program for violence prevention facilitators is available through trained staff at the RIPP office at Virginia Commonwealth University. This training follows the guidelines presented in Chapter 3 and includes a short evaluative consultation, as well as weekly consultation via e-mail during program start-up and implementation. Facilitators should participate in this training or something equally intensive so that your site adheres to the same guidelines. Costs for program materials are minimal and include RIPP instructor manuals (approximately $35 each), 3–4 violence prevention videos appropriate for students in your school, copying costs, pads of flip chart paper, a flip chart stand, markers, tape, folders for students, and index cards.

Once you have determined the costs, it is time to consider how to fund this program. Should the school hire new staff and completely run the program itself? Or should the school partner with another agency to run the program for the school? There are advantages either way. If the program belongs completely to the school, the school will have more control over using the resources for funding the program. However, the school may also get a lot of pressure to assign the program facilitator other tasks that will make it difficult for him or her to do the job well. For example, it may promote goodwill if a violence prevention facilitator supervises a classroom when a teacher is out sick, yet using facilitators this way regularly will prevent them from completing their own tasks. Partnering with another agency to facilitate the program for the school reduces the possibility that this will happen because the outside agency will determine the goals of the facilitator. It also cuts down on supervision and training costs and staffing because that will be the responsibility of the other agency. Having another agency involved, perhaps a public mental health center or a nonprofit agency that delivers prevention programs, may provide the opportunity for additional subsidiary services that they have available. Because collaboration is frequently required to assure grant funding, partnering might be beneficial to both the school and the agency.

If grants are the source of your funding for the RIPP program, be sure to plan ahead for sustainability. You might use grants to fund the early years of the program, intending that an evaluation of the program's success will convince the school board to allocate dollars to continue the program into the future. A program like RIPP takes a certain amount of time to really change the climate of the school. Keep future funding sources in mind as you begin to set up your program.

One way of ensuring sustainability is to develop advocates for the program from the beginning. Although the management team will be one group of such advocates, it is also their responsibility to increase this base of support. Forming a parent-community advisory committee might be one way of developing this advocacy by bringing together key parents and community leaders and exposing them to the goals and major components of the program. This will help to engage their assistance in thinking through ways of funding the program. You might also work with student leaders to create a marketing campaign within the school to develop support for RIPP. Explaining the program to the PTA at an early stage and securing their support for the program is another method of developing advocates. These advocates can be powerful voices to the school board when the decision of future funding is on the table.

LOGISTICS AND SUPERVISION

The logistics and supervision of the program will differ, depending on whether it is implemented in a single school or throughout a school system. If a systemwide program is the goal, you will have to lay a lot more groundwork than you would in a single school. In this case, it will be essential that the effort have the strong backing of administrators at the highest level.

As schools increasingly move to site-based management, each school is likely to have a different schedule and organizational structure. Deciding how the program will best fit into each school's schedule can happen only at the local level. You will have to spend time with each principal, ensuring his or her support and willingness to work to make the program a success. You will have to decide together where the program will be taught. One option is to work within a team and take one class from each major subject a month, rotating around the team each week. This will take a great deal of planning by the program coordinator and the principal but can be very effective because the whole team is exposed to the program and can better follow up by reminding the students of the basics taught in their classrooms. Another, and perhaps more common option, is to put the program in the health and physical education classroom. Yet another possibility is to use an extended homeroom period, if that exists in your school. There are a number of strategies for working this program into existing schedules; thinking creatively with principals and interested teachers will reveal many options. Creative thinking will also help determine ways to provide space for the violence prevention facilitator. In addition to classroom space for teaching the program, the facilitator will need a small office for planning and conducting peer mediations.

Another thing to consider is whether to phase in components of the program. For example, you might want to begin with the three curricula in the first year and add the peer mediation component in the following year. If your school is very large and there is a fair amount of doubt on the part of the faculty, you might want to consider a "pilot" year where you teach the curriculum to only half the students and measure the results against the comparison group (see Chapter 4 for details on conducting a pilot evaluation of RIPP). Another option may be to begin with the 6th grade curriculum only in the first year and add the 7th and 8th grade curricula in subsequent years.

Supervision and support for the violence prevention facilitator are extremely important to the success of the program. Because the RIPP facilitator is the only person in his or her school with that role, it will be important that he or she gain regular feedback and support. One component of this can be provided by having a meeting between the supervisor, the principal, and the facilitator at the beginning and end of the year to discuss the role and responsibilities of the facilitator at that school. Such a meeting can be used as a reference point if there are problems as the year progresses. It will be important for the RIPP facilitator to have regular opportunities for support and training throughout the school year. If RIPP is being implemented within a large school system, the RIPP facilitators can meet monthly; if RIPP is being implemented only at one school, the facilitator can join an already existing team of teachers/support staff for monthly meetings.

PEER MEDIATION

In addition to the curricula, peer mediation is a key element of the comprehensive RIPP program. Peer mediation is a program in which young people are trained to work in pairs to help students resolve their conflicts. Peer mediators use a technique in which they ask each student to tell his or her side of the story, ask them to describe how the conflict is making them feel, and then ask each party what they can do to resolve their participation in the conflict. It is a technique that is unique in several ways:

1. It assumes that there are at least two people who are responsible for what is happening and that there are very few conflicts in which one person does something bad to a totally innocent person. Both played a part in bringing the conflict about and both have to change some behavior to resolve it.
2. It assumes that students can resolve their own conflicts nonviolently. The fact that they use violent solutions is more a factor of environment and peer pressure or of not having learned the skills. Peer mediation is an example of empowering youth to solve problems.
3. By putting the responsibility on the students to resolve their own conflicts, peer mediation frees teachers to teach course material, rather than taking a lot of class time to solve the problem for the students.

The major purpose of having an official peer mediation program is that it provides an institutional affirmation that indeed there is a better way to resolve conflicts than resorting to power over other people—either the power of violence or the power of the administration. It is a way that school faculty and administration can send students the message that they have a real commitment to teaching the important life skill of appropriate conflict resolution. Fortunately, this education can be done without taking class time. Both peer mediators and those seeking mediation agree to be responsible for making up the work they miss while they are at mediation. Peer mediation integrates the school's commitment to nonviolence into the very structure of the school day in a public, visible way.

Peer Mediation and the Code of Discipline

Some school staff may express the concept that peer mediation could undermine the rules that have been established to make the school run smoothly and enable students to spend their day in a learning environment. On the contrary, peer mediation fits nicely into most codes of conduct. Because they do not have to spend lots of time dealing with conflicts, teachers can intervene early by recommending that students go to mediation at the first sign of trouble. Students may turn down this recommendation, and then if the conflict escalates, teachers would handle it the way they would handle any rule infraction. The hope—and experience of many schools who have used peer mediation—is that the conflict will be resolved and never escalate. Merely stopping a conflict rarely resolves it, and it usually pops up again later. The fight in the cafeteria at noon probably didn't start there; most likely it started small, early in the morning, or a day or two earlier.

If students fight and need to be suspended or whatever is called for by your code, mediation might be offered when the students return to school. Sending students home may teach them the consequences of violent behavior and can give them time to cool off, but it rarely actually resolves the conflict. Mediation upon return might do that, if the students agree.

Some infractions fall into a middle ground. Perhaps without the help of peer mediation, the teacher might have intervened with a disciplinary measure. Now, he or she might offer the students involved a choice: "I can take care of it by giving you a disciplinary referral, or you can go to peer mediation and solve it yourself."

Making sure that the violence prevention facilitator and the primary disciplinarian of the school are in close contact and agree on the parameters of the program is one way to ensure that there is no conflict between peer mediation and the code of discipline. There may be some trial and error attempts to integrate the two concepts, but if both trust and respect the other and recognize the importance of both elements in the school, the difficulties can be smoothly addressed. Mediation is for interpersonal conflicts between students. It does not work well with conflicts that students have with the institution—absenteeism, tardiness, or not abiding by school dress codes or other prohibitions. Ensuring that everyone is clear about what is most appropriate for mediation will go a long way toward making the referrals to mediation effective.

Confidentiality in Peer Mediation

Confidentiality is a key component of peer mediation. To gain the trust of the students agreeing to mediate their conflict, the mediators must guarantee that they will not discuss anything that goes on in the session with anyone else. The coordinator will be included in that bond of confidentiality, so that mediators can discuss a case with the coordinator if they are confused or need some clarity on how something was handled. The only thing that teachers or administrators are told is that the students in question came to mediation and whether they resolved their conflict. Many teachers want more than this; however, the integrity of the process requires that the interaction within the room be confidential. Teachers may want the resolution to pass their own internal criteria, but that is a standard to which the students cannot be held. It is more important that the students come to their own resolution.

Because some teachers and administrators may initially have trouble with this rule, it is important to lay the groundwork so that they understand its importance. Although the parties to the mediation cannot be held to the same rule of confidentiality because it is their conflict that is being resolved, most mediators will ask them not to discuss the details of the mediation or to tell private things that came up during the mediation. Some students may ask to have the confidentiality written into the agreement they reach with the other student, but even then there is no code requiring the other student to maintain that confidence. Our experience, however, is that most students have enough respect for the process they went through not to tell private things outside the room.

Peer mediators, on the other hand, should be bound strictly by the rules of confidentiality. Proof that a mediator has broken that rule should result in temporary suspension or dismissal as a peer mediator. In meetings where peer mediators are increasing their skills and getting help about difficult cases, names of mediating parties should never be used. If the situation is so obvious that everyone would know who it is, it should be discussed privately with the coordinator.

There is, of course, one area where confidentiality is not maintained, and that is anything that has to do with danger to either of the parties or to another student in the school. These may be revelations about child abuse, weapons, or drugs brought in to school. The students should be informed in advance that these topics are not covered by confidentiality and when something like that is brought up, the mediators should immediately get the coordinator.

Selection of Mediators

Choosing the most appropriate students to serve as peer mediators is crucial to the success of the program. These students must exhibit leadership and truly represent a cross section of the student body. If mediators represent only the most positive leaders in the school, those from other groups will not perceive that the process related to them. Even negative leaders should be chosen, because they can often convince a certain group of students to use the process. The diversity of the mediators should not be overlooked. In addition to the "groups" to which students belong, consider race, ethnicity, socioeconomic level, gender, and grade level. In addition to mediators who appeal to the diversity in the school, this diversity will also help students gain experience in dealing with students who are very different from them. You will not be making an effort to match students with specific mediators who look like them; however, the total group will be the proof that mediation is for everyone. In choosing the group, it is also a good idea to choose at least two students from each type or group. Participating in the training and becoming a mediator is a risk if it is new to the school, and being sure that no one is isolated or uncomfortable will help you keep the mediators longer.

You will want to look for personal leadership skills and ability to communicate well with others. Mediators should also demonstrate empathy and an ability to take feedback. Mediators can grow in their personal skills, but, especially in the first year of the program, you should look for real skill in the students that you choose. In addition to personal attributes, look for commitment to the program. Commitment can be determined by the students' willingness to participate in all parts of the training, their stated willingness to make up school work missed, their demonstrated participation in training, and their timeliness in making up school work.

It can be beneficial to have a few at-risk students as part of your pool. One of the greatest benefits of peer mediation is what happens to the mediators themselves. Besides learning valuable skills that can serve them in other avenues of their lives, mediators gain a certain stature in the school. For at-risk students, this opportunity frequently helps them channel the leadership skills they have been using negatively into positive activities. Although it may take a little more work on the part of the program coordinator to involve these at-risk students in the program, their experience with risky behaviors often makes their contributions very helpful to the whole program, once you have truly engaged them. Keep the power of positive peer pressure in mind when you select such students because you will want the majority of the students in peer mediation to be students who abide by school rules and are positive role models. Programs that have a majority of at-risk students in them perpetuate negative behaviors.

There are various ways to select mediators. The most effective approach is to poll the students with a simple question: "If you were to ask someone to help you resolve a conflict, who would you choose?" At the very least, you will get a good pool of students to choose from. You can then ask teachers to affirm these nominations. You should not solicit input only from teachers and administrators because that staff alone may not see the breadth of leadership you are looking for. It is important, however, for all staff to understand the requirements of diversity in creating a pool of mediators and to approve all of the students selected. If a teacher has strong reservations about any individual mediator, he or she can make it difficult for that student to participate by making it difficult for the student to make up work missed or by demanding perfection in all that the student does by way of "retaliation."

Training for Peer Mediation

There are many curricula to choose for training mediators. If you are choosing an outside agency to do the training, they will no doubt have their own training manual. We have included the names of several manuals in the bibliography; any of these will be adequate. It is important to involve someone in training who has had mediation experience. Teachers are accustomed to using a curriculum to teach concepts for which they do not have direct experience. In contrast, mediation is a skill that is difficult to teach if you have never been a mediator yourself. Even guidance counselors, who frequently think of themselves as mediators, are often so accustomed to being the ones who solve the problems or at least suggest solutions that they do not work well as mediation trainers, unless they have been specifically trained to do so.

You will need to find room in the schedule to allow adequate time for training mediators; most training models call for 16–18 hours of initial training. It is best to use two or three longer periods of time for the students to really get into the process. Using a Saturday with a couple of follow-up after-school sessions may work, though you may find that you are excluding students who cannot make it to the school building on Saturdays. An effective alternative is to find two school days when students can be released from classes and really have time to concentrate on the training. Such days may be most available at the beginning of the school year. The least effective alternative is to use a series of after-school sessions; students are tired at the end of the day, and the stopping and starting uses a lot of time getting the participants caught up and on target with the content. Although there is a great deal of evidence that students make excellent mediators, the skill of mediation is quite different from what most of them have experienced, and they need the full time to really understand their role and practice the skills. Do not skimp on training for the mediators and the teachers who will be working with them. The program will suffer if the students do not know what they are doing.

Logistics for Peer Mediation

Most training manuals help you make decisions about the logistics of running a peer mediation program. In fact, there are a number of books that discuss all of these points in great detail. The following are some of the key issues you should consider as you design your program.

One of the first issues is where the mediations will take place. Creative mediation programs have used spaces as small as a closet or as luxurious as a small office. The space needs to be large enough to hold a folding table and four chairs. There will need to be a locked file cabinet for the mediation report forms and other paperwork, though this could be located in the program facilitator's office. Another consideration about the space is whether you are going to require an adult to be present during the mediations. Many schools are nervous about leaving four students alone in a room for the mediation. It is our bias that this is the best method for student mediations, once the program facilitator has observed each peer mediator work through a conflict successfully. There should be an adult close by in case the mediators run into trouble, but there is no real need to have an adult in the room. In fact, students are more likely to be candid and honest if there is not an adult present.

The next decision is when mediations will be scheduled. Because peer conflict is not easily set aside in middle and junior high school, it is important to schedule the mediation closely after the referral. Scheduling mediations is the most complicated part of the process. There should be a central place where referrals are sent—a box in the library or the office. It should be easy for students and teachers to access and allow for at least some level of confidentiality. One way to make it happen is to schedule mediators throughout the day, depending on their schedules, for instance, scheduling mediators during a study hall or an elective class. Then the program facilitator can check the box every period, determine that the nature of the conflict is appropriate for peer mediation, and send for both the mediators and the disputants. Referrals made late in the day will be mediated the following day.

Another way to schedule mediations is for the program facilitator to look at each referral and put together a team of mediators that he or she feels would be most effective for these disputants. This method enables the coordinator to put together an effective team that mirrors the students asking for mediation in terms of skills, personality types, representation, etc. It takes more time and can be difficult when the schedule is hectic or unusual. There might also be a tendency for the coordinator to choose the same mediators again and again. This is not good for building the skill of the whole group of mediators.

Another decision concerns the best way to get the mediators and disputants into the same room together. If mediators are regularly scheduled, they can simply report to the mediation room during their assigned times and wait for potential disputants, or they can be called at the beginning of the period. Disputants should be given a slip that marks the time that they leave class and again the time that they leave the mediation session. This will prevent students from using extra time to get to and from class.

What about abuses? How can you know that students won't just manufacture disputes to get out of class? Of course, there are students everywhere who will find ways to use a system to their benefit. However, it has not been our experience that students abuse peer mediation. First of all, it would require a fair amount of coordination, because there are always two disputants involved. The program facilitator reviews the report forms regularly and if the same students were coming regularly for the same conflict, the facilitator might meet with the mediators involved to determine their evaluation of the sincerity of the efforts. The facilitator might then hold a meeting with the disputants to see if there is a problem that is making it necessary to mediate the same dispute again and again. This strategy is most likely to eliminate potential abuses.

There are many other details involved in setting up a peer mediation program that the consulting agency or the training manual will walk you through. There are several forms that need to be developed and kept. There is ongoing training and cohesion of the group of mediators. Setting up and running a peer mediation program requires attention to a myriad of details. However, careful attention to these details will pay off in improving the quality of the students' lives, as well as the quality of the school.

OBSTACLES TO IMPLEMENTING RIPP

What are some obstacles you might encounter in bringing RIPP to your school or system? Thinking through some of these will make the implementation less frustrating. One obstacle to be aware of is the ripple effect of changing a whole system to accommodate a new program, especially one as comprehensive as the RIPP program. Systems have lives of their own and adjust slowly to change, even change that represent improvements. You may encounter "turf" issues as students turn to another source to resolve their conflicts. Those who see their role diminishing may feel left out and may subtly begin to undermine the effectiveness of the system. Trying to think ahead about who those people might be and involving them from the beginning in program design and decisions will head off some of the problems. Another strategy is to guard against defensiveness when problems with initiating the program are introduced. Use the skills you have been developing as the initiator of an effective violence prevention program to model effective conflict resolution skills. Listening to those who have concerns will go a long way toward bringing them on board.

Another problem you might encounter, if you are doing a lot of different kinds of scheduling, is the program's impact on other extracurricular programs. You will not win any points for your program if you are not cooperative and are not a problem-solver as you work with the sponsors of other programs. Moreover, you may lose very good mediators if you require students to choose between mediation and other activities important to them.

Too frequently, schools initiate a new program, have a few meetings to familiarize teachers with this new innovation, and then expect the teachers to implement the program immediately. Sometimes it is a lack of funds for training. Sometimes it is the reality of the school situation whereby teachers work on a ten-month contract and planning additional training outside of that time is difficult. It is equally impossible to shut school down for several weeks while everyone is trained to do the new things.

To avoid these problems as you are planning your budget, keep in mind the importance of training the staff about the program (in addition to training the person responsible for implementing the program). There is a great deal of value in training as much of the staff as possible. If teachers do not understand the concepts taught in the RIPP curriculum, they could unintentionally undermine it. Students who are learning new ways to deal with interpersonal conflicts with other students will be more likely to inculcate the new ideas if they see them modeled and reinforced by teachers.

There are several ways to involve teachers in this training. One way is to devote in-service days to training the teachers. Another is to find funds to bring teachers in after school, on Saturdays, or during the summer to take the training. Teachers need to believe that young people can find a different way of resolving their conflicts and to understand the problem solving concepts taught by the program. They also need to find new ways to resolve the conflicts they have with each other and with students. If teachers continue to use disrespectful methods to resolve conflicts with students, students are not likely to believe that they can resolve their conflicts without violence. By disrespectful, we mean yelling or using sarcasm and demeaning language. We do not mean using appropriate consequences to discipline students who are out of order.

No matter how much training you do, there will still be those who are "unconverted." These teachers or other staff may have seen a number of programs come and go—each claiming it would change the world. They may be skeptical about the value of the RIPP program. All this work for another "flavor of the month" idea that will fade as quickly as the others. This is one reason to assure long-term survivability for RIPP. Being in it for the long haul will enable you to appeal to these staff members to wait and let the results speak for themselves. Another strategy that can be helpful is to have very clear objectives for the program, so that it is evident to all the staff exactly what the program can accomplish. A most helpful strategy is to try to anticipate who these "unconverted" are likely to be and engage them early in the process. That way they know they are being heard from the very beginning and will be less likely to hurl barbs when mistakes occur.

Another obstacle is fitting one more thing into a system filled with testing, accountability, and community report cards. Convincing teachers or administrators that there is room in the day for one more content area may be difficult. As we mentioned in the beginning of the chapter, if there is a need felt for less conflict during the school day, you may find your road easier. A careful examination of the RIPP curriculum in relation to the local standards of learning will help you make the connections. There is content in RIPP that fulfills the learning objectives in many communities. Being prepared with this information will help get administrators on board early with the program.

A final obstacle is the scheduling of standardized testing. The RIPP curriculum has been regularly revised to fit into the schedule of a school with a rigorous testing schedule. This means that the number of lessons that need to be taught over the course of the year allows for the fact that the class will not meet for certain periods of time. Program facilitators will have to be very flexible in implementing the program. Time is of the essence. The work described at the beginning of this chapter—building a network of support and getting teachers on board—will be especially important as you are trying to fit your program into the sometimes overwhelming demands of the system.

SUMMARY

What Works:

- Building a network of support from the beginning. These important people will help break the barriers that can loom large.
- Remember that it is the comprehensive nature of the program that truly makes it work. It is important to include all three curricula, the peer mediation program, and the corollary services of the coordinator or facilitator.

What Doesn't Work:

- Failure to be clear about what you think the program will accomplish will doom it from the beginning. People need to know that this program will affect the way students deal with their conflicts in school; it is not likely to change the face of violence in the city or country.
- Skimping on training for program staff and the staff and teachers at the school doesn't work. The more the concepts of RIPP are reinforced by the staff, the more likely they are to take root in the students.
- Failing to build a sustainable funding approach will jeopardize the program.
- Simply choosing teachers who are free to teach the program is a fatal error. The facilitators of the curriculum need to have a commitment to helping students really examine the role and effectiveness of violence in their lives. Assigning RIPP to a number of teachers because it seems they

could fit it in cannot build the commitment to change that the program requires.

What Might Work:

- There are alternatives to actually hiring new staff to teach the curriculum, but do it with care. Discern first the interest and level of commitment that teachers have to taking on this program.
- Phasing in the various components over a few years, while keeping the comprehensive picture in mind.

3

Selecting and Training
Beacons of Nonviolence

In this chapter, we describe the key issues related to selecting and training individuals to implement the RIPP program. As with all school-based health-promotion and social competence programs, adequate selection, preparation, and support of staff is essential. This chapter begins by defining the role of the prevention facilitator. Then, it describes some of the criteria for identifying individuals suited for this position. Finally, we provide an overview of the amount of time and type of activities required for training RIPP facilitators.

"BEACON OF NONVIOLENCE" DEFINED

The term "Beacon of Nonviolence" is used many times in this book to describe the violence prevention facilitator who implements the RIPP program. This term was chosen in the course of developing an interview protocol for recruiting of individuals to serve as violence prevention facilitators in an urban school system. The plan called for assigning one individual to serve in this role at each middle school in the school system. Beacon of nonviolence seemed to best describe the essence of this position and how a person in this role should operate, both inside and outside the school. We believed that these individuals should embody the power and principles of non-violence through their personal style and actions. This should be manifested through the way in which their teaching style facilitates student learning from the RIPP curriculum, through the way they model positive forms of conflict resolution with students and co-workers, and through the valued and influential role they hold in relationship to school administrators and the school community. In other words, the term "Beacon of Nonviolence" was used to describe clearly to interviewees how the person who implements the RIPP program must be willing to take on the responsibility of being a role model for nonviolence.

WHO IS THE VIOLENCE PREVENTION FACILITATOR?

The three primary components that determine who the violence prevention facilitator is and what he or she can do at each school are the role itself, the person who fulfills that role, and the way the person in that role fits in to the existing school structure. Our research and experience indicate that all three factors are equally important and highly interactive. For example, we have had experience with facilitators who could not get peer mediation programs initiated and could never fit into the school network. Whether this situation resulted from an ineffective facilitator, an unsupportive school network, or a combination of both, the end result was that students did not receive the program in its full form at these schools. Because of the importance of all three factors, this section will describe the role of the facilitator, criteria for selecting the facilitator, and strategies for optimizing the fit between the facilitator and a given school.

Simply stated, the responsibilities of the violence prevention facilitator are to teach RIPP to the 6th, 7th, and 8th grade classes weekly and to supervise and coordinate the peer mediation program. The 25-session RIPP-6 program is taught once a week for the entire year, beginning at the start of the school year; RIPP-7 is taught once a week for 12 weeks during the fall semester of the 7th grade year; and RIPP-8 is taught for 12 weeks during the spring semester of the 8th grade year. Depending on the size of the school and the number of students per grade, additional responsibilities can be added to reinforce RIPP and the peer mediation program. One example is to meet with students who have been suspended for fighting before they reenter the school. This meeting could be similar to a peer mediation session during which the facilitator makes sure the students have resolved their conflicts and helps them think through alternative methods for handling these conflicts in the future. Another example is to meet with student groups to identify any pockets of violence in the school and strategize about changing them. Other tasks might include working with teachers who are having problems with individual students to help them reinforce the concepts of RIPP, leading the crisis-response team, monitoring school lunches and bus loading/unloading, and conducting professional development seminars on conflict resolution for school staff.

Individuals hired to serve as prevention facilitators should have several important characteristics. To begin with, they should have a bachelor's degree in human services or a related field. They should also be committed to nonviolence and believe that aggression is not the only way for young people to resolve conflicts. There is an unspoken assumption among too many young people that a violent response is inevitable, that as much as they might want to resolve their conflicts in another way, it is not really possible. In fact, they may think that they are leaving themselves vulnerable if it seems that they do not want to fight. There is a great deal of violence in young people's lives these days—verbal violence if not always physical violence. Youth have precious few models for resolving conflicts in any other way. Even teachers, who hardly regard themselves as violent, may use intimidation to make things happen in their classrooms. For a young person this often translates into the lesson that, indeed, power over others is the only thing that works—and for too many of them power comes through violence, verbal or physical. Therefore, one of the most important qualities of the facilitator is to be a role model for the power of nonviolence that students can emulate. The facilitator must be willing to search within himself or herself to identify personal issues around power and to examine the depth of his or her own commitment to nonviolence. This commitment should show up in the examples that the facilitator brings to the teaching of the curriculum and in interactions with the class and with other faculty and administrators. The facilitator should be a "beacon of nonviolence" in the school whose modeling reflects the goals of the RIPP program. Whereas such an attitude may not be evident during the interview, a willingness to participate in training to facilitate such self-discovery is necessary. From our own experience, we have found that such training, combined with the realization of what today's youth are actually exposed to, is critical in developing facilitators who can speak convincingly to young people about the value and power of nonviolence.

It is also important to select individuals who will serve as a "facilitator," not a "director" in the classroom. Although many newer teachers coming into the classroom have been taught this approach, for years teachers were taught to be directors; they had the content they wanted the students to learn and whether it related to the students' experiences was irrelevant. The RIPP curriculum is a facilitated curriculum; each lesson tries to take the students' life experiences and draw on them to help them experience the possibilities of nonviolent alternatives. Many programs teach conflict resolution without first addressing students' experiences of violence. In using this approach, one often meets with an unstated resistance. Students instinctively know that resolving conflicts is not always possible, and unless the program teaches them a variety of techniques for dealing with their problems, they are not likely to believe that resolution is possible, even in those circumstances where it is the best method. Thus, being able to facilitate the participants' ability to get in touch with their own experiences and reflect on them to determine results and consequences is critical to teaching the RIPP curriculum. Prevention facilitators should also have excellent public speaking and presentation skills; a dynamic presentation of material enhances the possibility that students will pay attention to what is being taught.

The RIPP program is highly experiential; students are provided with role-plays and other experiences that help them to simulate real life circumstances in which they might have to use these new methods. As anyone who has ever tried it knows, experiential education means that students are up and out of their seats as they work on the concepts being covered. Therefore, facilitators must be comfortable with a certain amount of apparent confusion in the classroom setting. This person must be able to maintain control without some of the more external signs of control—students at their desks working quietly. In other words, they need to have excellent classroom management skills.

Prevention facilitators must also be committed to youth empowerment. Whereas most educators would express such a commitment, really understanding and having a commitment to youth empowerment is critical to the success of the RIPP program. The facilitator must believe that these young people have it within themselves to make the right choices in spite of what they may be witnessing around them. To believe in youth empowerment is to turn decisions over to the participants in the class whenever possible. To empower youth within a classroom setting and still keep control of the curriculum and of the class is a delicate task. It requires a facilitator with a strong sense of self and a willingness to live a commitment to the value of conflict resolution and violence prevention.

Another side of this role of "Beacon of Nonviolence" is to be willing to promote the program. Because the RIPP program will be new and subject to preconceived notions about programs that come and go, the RIPP facilitator will need to learn how school personnel feel about outsiders and prepare a plan of action. Consultations with the management team will be extremely important in this process. Another important component will be to generate discussions with staff about youth violence and what nonviolence means to them. Such discussions will open a line of communication between the program facilitator and school staff regarding what can be done to improve the school climate.

Finally, prevention facilitators must have demonstrated their ability to work collaboratively with a team because they will need to work closely with all school staff. A person who can market himself or herself to the school staff and clearly demonstrate the value of his or her role will find it easier to fit in. Again, all of the things we said about being a model for resolving conflicts will come into play. Another way to enhance the fit between the facilitator and the school setting is to have the principal involved in the interview and selection process for this person. We have found this especially helpful when an interview pool does not include qualified candidates who fit the demographics desired by the principal. For example, in our urban school system where 96% of the student population is African-American, there is high demand for male African-American school staff and most schools want their violence prevention facilitator to be an African-American male. When principals are involved in the interview process, they can look beyond the characteristics of ethnicity and gender to consider a bigger picture about which person would be the best match for their school. Because we include principals in the interview process and because principals are likely to support the goals of the RIPP program, they are often the strongest advocate for the facilitator in the school.

WE'VE HIRED GREAT PEOPLE WILLING TO TAKE ON THIS RESPONSIBILITY—NOW WHAT?

Once a qualified individual has been hired to promote nonviolence, training must be provided to facilitate the transformation of potential into actuality. Because prevention facilitators may come from a wide range of educational backgrounds, varying strengths will be brought to the table. For example, a person who has a background in education is likely to have a stronger base of skills in classroom management and presentation than a person with a background in social work, who may have a stronger base in interpersonal skills and strategies for dealing with crises. If more than one person is being trained, such diversity in educational background can serve to enrich the training experience. This diversity may provide a challenge to a trainer, however, who must work to bring participants to relatively high levels of competence across multiple areas.

Although there are many topics that need to be covered in training, they fall into three main categories that need to be covered to prepare each staff person who is going to implement RIPP. The first category, Training in Ways to Promote Nonviolence and in Experiential Education, provides a base for the rest of the training and requires approximately four days (32 hours). The second category, Training in Program Objectives and RIPP Curriculum, provides specific training in program content and issues related to early adolescence. For RIPP-6, this requires approximately four days (32 hours). If a person has already been trained in RIPP-6, training for RIPP-7 and RIPP-8 each require two days (16 hours); if a person has not been trained in RIPP-6, the training time for RIPP-7 and RIPP-8 increases to four days for each (32 hours). The third category, Training in Peer Mediation, requires at least one day a year, each year. Ongoing training throughout the year in additional topics, such as crisis response and stress management are also important, but are not part of the core training for RIPP. These are discussed briefly at the end of this chapter.

Overview of Training

The goal of training is for participants to leave well prepared for their violence prevention role—we call this "training for competence." For that reason, the training sessions are comprised of many opportunities for self-reflection, practice, and feedback. The following represents an outline of the content of the various components of training.

Promoting Nonviolence

- Understanding the Positive and Negative Sides of Power
- Relationships as the Key to Change
- Active Listening and I-messages
- Language and Violence
- Understanding Nonviolence
- Differences/Diversity
- Team-Building
- Local, National, and Global News

Experiential Education

- World Views of Education
- The Experiential Learning Cycle
- Facilitation Skills
- Establishing Ground Rules
- Using Small Groups
- Role-Playing

Training in RIPP Objectives

- Prevention/Health Promotion (vs. Intervention)
- Developmental Tasks in Early Adolescence
- Nonviolence During Early Adolescence
- The 12 RIPP Objectives

Training in Program Content and Implementation

- RIPP-6
- RIPP-7
- RIPP-8
- Peer Mediation
- Presentation Skills (eye contact, voice, body language, handling questions)
- Classroom Management

Ongoing Training

During the school year, it is important to provide opportunities for staff development and training for RIPP facilitators. Additional topics that can be covered include one-on-one case management, crisis response, passive restraint, how to conduct staff development training, what works and what does not work in small, pull-out groups, and stress management. Experts who can conduct such training are available in most communities, through church groups, educational consortiums, and the like.

Coping with Staff Changes

One of the realities of the professional world is that staff changes occur after training has been completed. For that reason, it is important for the management team to have procedures in place for coping with such changes. When new staff are hired, a buddy-mentor relationship can be developed between senior staff and new staff. If your program is at just one school and there are no other staff with whom to partner, consider expending a few resources to have your new staff member "shadow" a RIPP staff member in another school system. The Life Skills Center keeps track of schools that are implementing RIPP and may be able to help identify a nearby school.

SUMMARY

What Works:

- Choosing your program facilitators with care. These are the "Beacons of Nonviolence" against which the early stages of the program will be measured.
- Training by Life Skills Center staff.
- On-going training throughout the year.

What Doesn't Work:

- Skimping on training.

What Might Work:

- Consulting with RIPP Project staff to develop your own training.
- Utilizing local experts.

4

Knowing whether RIPP Is Working in Your School

OVERVIEW

This chapter is designed to help individuals implementing the RIPP program determine whether it is producing its desired effects. Although many books conclude with a chapter about evaluation, we placed this chapter closer to the beginning because we believe that it is important to think about evaluation from the very beginning. Too often, evaluation is an afterthought. When this happens, evaluation is likely to be viewed as burdensome, as opposed to something that will improve the entire project. Our hope is that placing this chapter directly after training and before the program descriptions will increase the chance that efforts to prevent youth violence will include a fully integrated evaluative component.

This chapter begins by arguing for the importance of incorporating some level of evaluation into every implementation of RIPP. Then, we outline some of the initial steps needed to prepare for an evaluation, including putting together an evaluative team. This is followed by a discussion of different evaluative models and some key issues related to evaluative design. We conclude by recommending the minimum elements that should be incorporated into any evaluation of RIPP.

WHY IS EVALUATION SO IMPORTANT?

Because previous evaluations found evidence to support the effectiveness of RIPP, some readers may question why it is necessary to continue to evaluate it. Couldn't the resources required to conduct an evaluation be better used for other purposes? There are several reasons why continued evaluation of RIPP (or any prevention program) is well worth the effort and expense involved. Local evaluation is necessary to help those involved in implementing the program determine if it is meeting its objectives, to provide accountability to various stakeholders, to ensure that the program is correctly implemented, and to provide a basis for its continual improvement. This is often referred to as "empowerment evaluation" (Fetterman, 1996).

In Chapter 2, we discussed the importance of developing school-level goals and short-term objectives that reflect the things that staff would like to see change as a result of implementing the RIPP program. Once these goals are established and a plan of action is implemented, the logical next step is to determine if the program is having its desired effects. After all, the most critical goal is not to implement a violence prevention program, but to address specific problems at a particular school. Implementing a violence prevention program should be seen as a means to an end, rather than an end in and of itself. Although the RIPP program was effective in meeting many of the goals of the school systems where it has been implemented thus far, other schools or school systems may identify different goals they would like to see addressed by this program. Conducting a local evaluation is the only way to clearly establish if such goals are being met. If implementation of a program does not address all of the program's objectives, other methods of addressing those objectives may need to be considered.

Evaluation findings may also be needed to document the program's impact for various stakeholders. Stakeholder is a term used in evaluation research to describe those that are affected either directly or indirectly by the results of an evaluation (Fetterman, 1996; Rossi & Freeman, 1993). For the RIPP program, such stakeholders might include school superintendents, school board members, and others responsible for deciding whether the program should be implemented; agencies that provide funds for program implementation; school staff and administrators that support the program's implementation; the prevention facilitators who implement it; the students who participate in it; the parents of these students; and other members of the community. Evaluating the impact of a program will be of considerable interest to those involved in its implementation. Prevention facilitators, in particular, will want to know whether what they are doing is "making a difference." Although their own informal observations may provide some indication of their overall effectiveness, more formal methods of evaluation will provide more objective evidence of program effects. As with other programs, successful implementation of RIPP requires a high level of support from a variety of stakeholders. Evidence that supports program effectiveness may be critical to maintaining such support. In cases where evaluation evidence indicates that the program is not meeting its goals, this information may be critical in convincing decision-makers to implement changes in the program or to introduce a different program altogether. Such decisions help empower the community where the program is being implemented (Fetterman, 1996). For example, we used evaluation findings to justify developing the RIPP program, using it to replace an existing violence prevention program, expanding it from 14 to 25 sessions, and extending the program into all three middle school grades.

The effectiveness of implementing RIPP in a new setting should not be assumed. Our previous evaluations of RIPP found that certain desirable outcomes (e.g., changes in disciplinary code violations) were obtained when several prevention facilitators implemented the RIPP program with a particular population of students within a particular context. Although this specific mix of program ingredients led to desirable outcomes, this process needs to be replicated to determine whether similar results can be obtained under other conditions. For example, the primary evaluation study of RIPP-6 was conducted in the urban schools using prevention facilitators who all happened to be African-American men, most of whom had several previous years of experience implementing other violence prevention programs within the same schools. Whether their race, gender, previous experience, and/or other characteristics they may have had in common were critical to the success of the program remains unknown. Similarly, the impact of the program has been examined in two very different settings—with a largely African-American sample of students in an urban school system and with a more ethnically diverse sample of students at a rural school. Will RIPP produce similar effects in suburban schools, private schools, schools located in other regions, larger schools, smaller schools, or schools that serve a different combination of grades (i.e., junior high versus middle school configurations)? How important is the match between the prevention facilitators and the student population? Would RIPP have produced the same effect in the urban schools if it had been implemented by Caucasian or female prevention facilitators? The answers to these and other similar questions can be determined only by continued replication and evaluation of the program's impact.

Integrating evaluation into every implementation of RIPP is also necessary to ensure that the program is implemented correctly. Prior to developing RIPP, we conducted an evaluation of another school-based program (Farrell & Meyer, 1997). Our evaluation of this program indicated that prevention facilitators showed considerable variability in how they interpreted the curriculum and implemented the program. In developing the RIPP training materials, we made every effort to provide clear instructions and examples to facilitate more consistency in implementing the program across different prevention facilitators. Providing such materials is, however, no guarantee that they will be followed. In our evaluations of RIPP, we include process observations (i.e., actual observations of the way the program is being implemented) that enable us to determine whether all of the major components of the curriculum are followed. If other implementations of RIPP do not adhere to these practices, they may be more or less effective.

At this point it is unclear which elements must be faithfully reproduced and which may be modified to "fine-tune" RIPP for a particular setting. For example, because the original RIPP program was developed within the context of a school system that served a predominantly African-American student population, many of the examples and curriculum materials such as videotapes were selected for relevancy to this population. When this program was implemented with a more ethnically diverse student population in rural schools, some modifications were made to make the program more appropriate for that population (see Chapter 8). Evaluation of any new implementation of RIPP is critical to accurately describe which program elements were faithfully replicated and which were modified and to determine the extent to which the program was effective. Such work will ultimately provide a basis for determining the most effective combination of program components for a given student population and setting.

All of the preceding reasons for integrating evaluation into the implementation of RIPP share a common goal of providing a basis for continually improving the program's effectiveness. This strategy is an integral part of an action-research model in which evaluation findings provide a basis for continually refining and improving the program. The original development of RIPP was guided by this action-research approach (see Chapter 1), and this approach is critical to its continued development as it is implemented in other communities. We believe that such an approach will ultimately lead to the identification of the specific strategies and combinations of strategies that work best with specific populations. Such evaluation findings also provide a basis for continually improving effectiveness. For example, if referrals for peer mediation are particularly low at some schools and particularly high at others, sharing information about the way the program is implemented across different schools can help identify factors that may increase participation in the program. Although the current RIPP program produces a number of desirable outcomes, to implement it in a new community without conducting an evaluation assumes that it will produce positive benefits and also that it cannot be improved. Integrating evaluation into each implementation of RIPP will ensure that we are continually challenged to improve the effects of our interventions.

ASSEMBLING AN EVALUATION TEAM

One of the first steps in conducting an evaluation of RIPP is to assemble an evaluation team. Members of this team will provide the necessary expertise to conduct a systematic evaluation of a local implementation of RIPP. This chapter provides an overview of some of the important issues involved in conducting an evaluation of RIPP. It is not, however, intended to provide a step-by-step guide to conducting an evaluation, nor does it provide a sufficient basis for training someone unfamiliar with evaluation methodology to conduct such an evaluation. The most appropriate design for evaluating any given implementation of RIPP will depend on a variety of factors, including the setting, the goals of the implementation, the characteristics of the students, and a variety of practical considerations. A properly trained evaluation expert or team is needed to determine the most appropriate design for a given application, to conduct the statistical analyses, and interpret the findings. Individuals with such expertise may be found in some school systems, within state agencies, at local universities, and in private consulting firms.

Some of the factors to consider in selecting evaluators include their expertise in evaluation methodology and statistical methods, experience evaluating prevention programs and working in school settings, and familiarity with outcome measures appropriate for evaluating a violence prevention program. It is also important to find individuals willing to work as part of a team within the context of the action-research model described previously. Such evaluators do not simply make judgments about whether or not a given program is effective, but are committed to using the findings from an evaluation to guide efforts to improve the effectiveness of the intervention.

The evaluation plan should be based on sound evaluation principles, be consistent with the goals of the program, and the tailored to the specific school settings. For this reason, it is extremely important that the individuals responsible for conducting the evaluation work closely with the management team (see Chapter 2). This will ensure that they have a thorough understanding of the intervention and its goals and access to individuals who are familiar with the particular schools that participate in the evaluation. Excluding any one group of individuals is unlikely to result in a plan that meets each of these objectives. The management team can also help troubleshoot problems that may arise during the evaluation and can provide a useful perspective for interpreting the evaluation findings.

LAYING THE GROUNDWORK

Successfully completing an evaluation of a school-based program such as RIPP requires the support of stakeholders and other individuals who will be asked to participate in the evaluation. Lack of support at even one level can be sufficient to block the completion of a successful evaluation. The approval of some central administrative authority (e.g., superintendents, school board members) may be needed before individual schools can be approached to participate in the evaluation process. School principals may be asked to provide data for the evaluation (e.g., disciplinary referrals), and assistance in scheduling implementation and evaluation activities. Teachers may be asked to give up instructional time so that students can participate in the intervention and evaluation activities (e.g., completing surveys), to complete measures on their students, and more generally to promote the importance of these activities to the students. The cooperation of students is needed in participating in the program and completing any evaluation instruments. Depending on the evaluation design, parents may also be asked to provide data on their children or to approve their participation in some activities (e.g., interviews, focus groups). This section discusses some of the key concerns and issues that may be encountered when prevention programs are evaluated in school settings. Addressing these issues is critical to conducting a successful evaluation.

Those asked to participate in an evaluation are unlikely to give their full cooperation if they do not appreciate its value. The very use of the term evaluation may raise concerns about who or what is being evaluated. School officials, principals, teachers, prevention facilitators, students, and parents may be concerned that the evaluation will in some way reflect negatively on their performance. One approach that has been helpful in addressing this concern is to clarify that the focus is on evaluating or improving the effectiveness of the program, not the individuals responsible for implementing it, the sites where it is conducted, or the students who participate. Those involved in conducting an evaluation of RIPP might suggest that the program has been effective elsewhere, but that we need to see how well it works for us and whether we can improve it. Our own efforts to evaluate RIPP within the urban public school system have been successful to a large extent because of the high level of cooperation between the school staff and the evaluation team. During the eight years of this project, there has been a growing appreciation of the benefits of the evaluation work we have conducted. Each year the evaluation results have been used to guide changes in the program that led to increases in its effectiveness. Evidence of the effectiveness of the program, in turn, has facilitated obtaining continued funding for the program, pride in contributing to a larger national effort to address youth violence, and recognition for the program itself. Such an appreciation may develop gradually, and others involved in implementing and evaluating RIPP should not be discouraged if there is less than enthusiastic support for their initial evaluative efforts.

It is also important to address concerns about the way the data collected for evaluation will be used and to whom it will be reported. School officials may be concerned that data on the frequency of violent behavior within their schools may be reported by the press and used to reflect negatively on their schools. Principals may be concerned that such data may be used to make comparative statements about different schools (e.g., Which school is the most violent?). At a more general level, teachers and others may be concerned that such data may be used to represent their students in a poor light. For example, teachers in a school system that serves a predominantly minority population may be concerned that data may be used to portray these students as "bad kids." Finally, students may be concerned that reporting their involvement in violence or other problem behavior will get them in trouble.

In our experience, the best way to address these concerns is to confront them directly. We worked with the school system to develop a clear policy regarding the way data would be reported. Such a policy should address the types of data that would be reported and the outlet for such reports, the smallest unit for which data would be reported (e.g., at the school system rather than individual school level), and when the specific school system will be identified in publications. Addressing teachers' concerns involves clarifying the purpose of collecting evaluation data and the way it will be used. Student concerns need to be addressed by providing a clear statement regarding the procedures that will be used to protect their confidentiality. More will be said about this later in our discussion of data collection procedures. The basic issue is often one of trust. We have found that many of these concerns have diminished over time. Still, however, we occasionally encounter a teacher who actively discourages students from providing data.

One method that we have found effective in generating support for the collection of evaluation data has been to help the schools use these data for other purposes. We routinely provide each principal at schools that participate in a RIPP evaluation with a report that summarizes student responses to each item in our evaluation battery and examines changes over time. Principals are told that they may use these reports for their own purposes and that we will not report this information to others (i.e., each principal sees a report based on their own school). Principals and administrative staff have shown considerable interest in these reports and have used them for their own planning purposes. We have also honored requests for analyses to address questions of special interest to particular principals. For example, we have prepared reports that compare one wing of the school to the other, examine trends across grades, and examine changes in a specific grade across cohorts. We have also provided reports to the school system that have been used for planning and to provide descriptive data to support the applications for various types of funding. This has helped develop an appreciation for the value of collecting these data and has demonstrated that the flow of information is not a one-way street.

A final step in preparing for an evaluation involves obtaining the necessary approval from an appropriate institutional review board. This approval is needed to grant permission to conduct the evaluation and also to review the procedures to be employed to make certain that they fall within appropriate ethical guidelines and that they protect the rights of all participants. Although most evaluation teams can be expected to follow ethical guidelines, an independent review by a duly appointed committee provides a system of checks and balances to ensure that all relevant ethical issues are considered and may be necessary to satisfy specific legal requirements. Most universities, state agencies, and large school systems have standing committees established to evaluate any research or evaluation studies. Care must always be taken to protect the rights of individuals who participate in evaluation studies. Several professional organizations including the American Psychological Association (American Psychological Association, 1992) and American Evaluation Association (Shadish, Newman, Scheirer, & Wye, 1995) have published guidelines that address relevant ethical issues. Specific federal guidelines related to the protection of research subjects may also apply (Office for Protection From Research Risks, 1991). Whether these guidelines are applicable depends upon a variety of factors, including whether the evaluation is considered to be research, the setting in which it is conducted, and the procedures that are used to obtain data. Individuals responsible for conducting an evaluation should be familiar with these guidelines and consult with a review board even when a project appears to be exempt from regulations.

TYPES OF EVALUATIONS

Evaluation studies of prevention programs such as RIPP are likely to employ different designs and methods, depending upon their specific focus. Figure 4.1 depicts a simple model that describes the mechanism by which RIPP is expected to produce its effects. According to this model, implementation of RIPP is expected to produce specific changes in the knowledge, attitudes, and behaviors targeted by the program. These changes in proximal outcomes are, in turn, expected to produce changes in more distal outcomes related to the longer term objectives of the program such as reducing incidents of physical fighting, weapons carrying, and fight- related injuries. A complete evaluation of RIPP involves examining each step in this model.

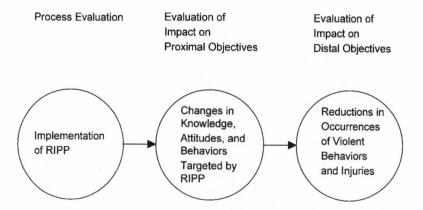

Figure 4.1. Model for evaluating RIPP. According to this model, implementation of RIPP is expected to produce specific changes in the knowledge, attitudes, and behaviors targeted by the program. These changes in proximal outcomes are, in turn, expected to produce changes in more distal outcomes related to the longer term objectives of the program such as reducing incidents of physical fighting, weapons carrying, and fight-related injuries.

Process Evaluations

There is little value in determining the effectiveness of an intervention if it is not possible to describe how the intervention was implemented. In other words, it is hard to evaluate something if you do not know *what* you are evaluating. Conducting a process evaluation of a program provides information that can be extremely valuable in interpreting outcome findings. If a local evaluation of RIPP indicates that it was not effective, this may mean that it didn't work with that specific target population or that it was not properly implemented. Numerous factors can interfere with the successful implementation of a program. For example, the prevention facilitators may not have the necessary qualifications or training to implement it, they may not faithfully adhere to the standardized implementation procedures described in the manual, the implementation schedule may result in the exclusion of many students, or the program may not have the adequate support of school staff. The extent to which such factors may have influenced the outcome of an evaluation cannot be determined if they are not assessed. Moreover, documenting differences in the procedures used to implement the program across evaluations provides a basis for determining the conditions necessary to produce change and also the conditions that improve the program's effectiveness.

A variety of approaches may be used to evaluate the implementation of RIPP. These include documenting the criteria used to select prevention facilitators, their qualifications, and the procedures used to train them. A process evaluation also involves collecting basic information such as how many students participated in the program, how many sessions they participated in, and how many students were excluded and why. Evaluations should also include an assessment of program fidelity, or the extent to which the key elements of the curriculum, as spelled out in the manual, are adhered to. In our own evaluations of RIPP, we have had observers sit in the back of the classroom, complete a checklist of the key elements for each lesson, and record any events that may have influenced the implementation. When this is not possible, it may be helpful to ask the prevention facilitators to complete these checklists. These data are obviously less objective, but they may provide useful information about the implementation process. Finally, interviews with school administrators, teachers, and focus groups of students may be conducted to assess the degree of support for the program within the school and to generate suggestions for improving its effectiveness.

Outcome Evaluations

Studies designed to assess the impact of prevention programs such as RIPP should focus on both proximal or immediate outcomes, as well as more distal or long term objectives (see Figure 4.1). Studies of proximal outcomes evaluate the specific areas that an intervention was designed to address. In other words, did the participants learn what the intervention was designed to teach them? For example, RIPP participants are expected to demonstrate increased knowledge of the material covered in the curriculum, to develop attitudes that are more favorable toward the use of nonviolent methods of resolving conflict, and to demonstrate specific skills addressed in the program such as *resolve, avoid, ignore,* and *diffuse.* Studies of distal outcomes focus on the longer term objectives that an intervention was designed to address. Because the long-term objective of RIPP is to reduce a participants' involvement in violence, as either victims or perpetrators, studies of distal outcomes would be expected to focus on violent behaviors.

Unlike process evaluations, which are largely descriptive, outcome or impact studies require the use of evaluation designs that enable the evaluator to examine change and also to make inferences about the factors responsible for those changes. For example, an evaluator might note a decrease in fighting among 6th graders who participated in RIPP-6. Does this mean that RIPP was responsible for this decrease? This question cannot be answered without additional data. Perhaps some other change within the school (e.g., changes in staff, stronger enforcement of disciplinary policies) or community (e.g., parents spending more time discussing nonviolence with children based on local or national events such as school shootings) was responsible for this decrease. For this reason, impact studies typically involve some comparison group or control group that can help isolate the effects of an intervention. Issues related to designing and implementing outcome studies are addressed in the following section.

In conclusion, conducting a comprehensive evaluation of a prevention program such as RIPP involves three separate steps. A process evaluation is necessary to document that the intervention was successfully implemented and to detail any local modifications that may have been required. Although it has been suggested that a thorough process evaluation may be sufficient when replicating effective programs, our current state of knowledge regarding effective violence prevention programs is too limited to support such an approach (see reviews by Catalano, Berglund, Ryan, Lonczak, & Hawkins, 1998; Elliott & Tolan, 1999; Samples & Aber, 1998). Few programs have been rigorously evaluated, and considerable work is needed to establish the conditions under which each program can be expected to be effective. More specifically, although the results of our evaluations of RIPP have been encouraging, it would be foolhardy to assume that this program will be equally effective everywhere it might be used.

Thus, school systems that implement RIPP are encouraged to employ the full evaluation model depicted in Figure 4.1. Results of the process evaluation will clarify which procedures were faithfully executed and which were modified to accommodate local conditions. This may serve as a useful starting point during the first year of implementing RIPP. Evaluations of the impact on proximal outcomes will indicate which program objectives are being successfully achieved and which are not. Such information can be used to improve the effectiveness of the curriculum by identifying areas that may need to be addressed in greater depth. Evaluations of distal outcomes will determine the extent to which the program is meeting its overall objectives. The greatest gains will come from integrating the findings of all three approaches. Such an integration will provide a basis for determining the effectiveness of RIPP as it is implemented across a variety of conditions, identifying modifications that improve its effectiveness, and providing a basis for designing the optimum intervention for a specific target population and setting.

EVALUATION DESIGNS

This section discusses some of the decisions that need to be made to conduct an evaluation of a prevention program such as RIPP. Developing an evaluation design involves deciding who will participate in the evaluation, the conditions to which they will be assigned, and the method that will be used to assign them to conditions. Evaluators must also be careful in selecting measures that are appropriate to the target population and that reflect the goals of the intervention. As this section shows, each of these decisions must be made with care because they have important implications for drawing conclusions about the effectiveness of the intervention being evaluated. This section is intended to provide an overview of these issues. Readers interested in a more general discussion of relevant methodological issues should refer to the excellent sources available on evaluation methodology (e.g., Chen, 1990; Cook, Anson, & Walchli, 1993; Rossi & Freeman, 1993) and prevention research (Bryant, Windle, & West, 1997). More specific information about strategies for evaluating school-based violence prevention programs may be found in Farrell, Meyer, Kung, and Sullivan (in press).

Selecting Treatment Conditions

Designs evaluating the effectiveness of prevention programs usually involve assigning participants to various groups, typically referred to as treatment conditions. A common design for evaluating RIPP includes a treatment group that participates in RIPP and a no-treatment control group that does not. The control group provides a basis for determining the impact of the intervention by showing what would have been likely to happen to members of the treatment group if they had not participated in the program. The absence of a comparison group makes it impossible to draw reasonable conclusions about the impact of a prevention program. For example, if students who participated in a prevention program showed an increase in violent behavior, one might initially conclude that the program was not effective. In fact, it may be that the program was effective in preventing a

larger increase from occurring. An example of such a finding from one of our own
evaluation studies of RIPP is reported in Figure 4.2. This figure indicates that
disciplinary code violations for carrying weapons increased from 0.5% to 1.0%
among students who participated in RIPP-6. It would be difficult to interpret this
as a success in the absence of any other data. Further examination of this figure,
however, indicates that the rate increased from 0.4% to 4.2% among students who
did participate in RIPP-6. In this instance the control group provides a basis for
concluding that the program was effective in reducing the increase in weapons
carrying.

Evaluation designs that assign some students to a no-treatment control group
are rarely greeted with enthusiasm by school officials and other concerned parties
who may be hesitant to withhold what they perceive as an effective intervention
from those they believe could benefit from it. It may also be difficult to recruit
schools to participate in an evaluation if there is a chance that they will be assigned to a no-treatment control condition. Nonetheless, as the preceding example
illustrates, it may be impossible to evaluate the impact of an intervention without
such a group. A possible compromise may be to stagger the implementation of the

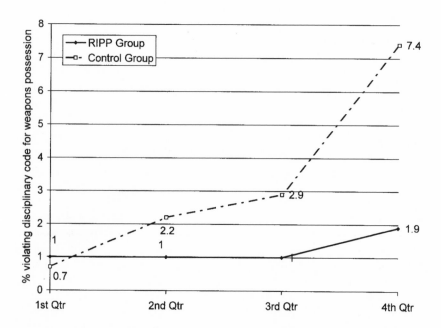

Figure 4.2. Example showing the importance of including a control group. This evaluation of
RIPP shows that the prevalence of disciplinary code violations for bringing weapons to schools
increases for students who participated in RIPP and students in a no-intervention control group.
The increase, however, was significantly greater among students who did not participate in RIPP.

program so that some students receive it before others. We employed just such a design in evaluating another violence prevention program (see Farrell & Meyer, 1997). Within this design, approximately half of the students participated in the intervention in the fall semester, the other half during the spring semester, and data were collected at the beginning, middle, and end of the school year. The midpoint assessment provided a basis for examining program effects by comparing students who had participated in the program during the fall semester to those that had not yet started the program. Although this design satisfied the school system's requirement that all 6th graders participate in the program, it had several shortcomings. In particular, we could not evaluate the longer term impact of the program.

The addition of other treatment conditions to an evaluative design can provide a basis for comparing the relative effectiveness of different prevention programs and identifying the factors that improve program effectiveness. For example, a school system that is attempting to choose between RIPP and some other prevention program could conduct a comparative study in which some students are assigned to each program. The outcome of such a study would indicate which program was most effective in their setting. The impact of supplementing RIPP with other prevention efforts can also be examined. For example, students could be assigned to three conditions: (1) a no-treatment control group, (2) a group that participates in RIPP, and (3) a group that participates in RIPP plus some supplementary program designed to strengthen its effects (e.g., after school program, teacher training, parent training). A further possibility is to evaluate the extent to which different methods of implementing RIPP influence its effectiveness. In such a design, the evaluator might systematically vary the conditions under which different groups of students participate in RIPP and examine differences in outcomes for such groups. Such evaluations could examine the relative effectiveness of using health educators rather than prevention facilitators to implement the program, or implementing the program on a more intensive schedule over a shorter period of time versus once a week throughout the year.

Assigning Students to Conditions

Once the treatment conditions have been identified, the next step in designing an impact evaluation is to identify which students will be assigned to the treatment conditions and determine how they will be assigned to specific conditions. As a primary prevention program, RIPP was designed to be implemented with the majority of middle school students. Practical considerations related to scheduling (e.g., students not taking physical education class if that is the class designated for implementation of the program) might also prevent some students from participating in a RIPP evaluation. Evaluations should document which students are not assigned to treatment conditions and the reasons for their exclusion to identify clearly the sample that participates in the evaluation. This is important because students should be actively assigned to each treatment condition, not simply assigned by default. For example, if all students at a school who don't participate in RIPP are considered the control group, this group could include students who were screened from participation in the program for various reasons. Such students should be screened out of both treatment conditions, so that they do not bias either group (e.g., having all the high-risk children end up in the control group).

Strategies for assigning students to treatment conditions typically fall into two categories—within-school designs and between-school designs. Within-school designs involve assigning students within each school to every treatment condition. For example, half of the students in each school are assigned to the intervention group and half to the control group. Students may be assigned to conditions as individuals, based on their homeroom period or the team of teachers to whom they are assigned. Between-school designs involve assigning entire schools to treatment conditions. For example, RIPP might be implemented with all students at five schools assigned to the treatment condition and five other schools assigned to a no-treatment control condition.

Between-school and within-school designs each have distinct advantages and disadvantages for evaluating prevention programs (Farrell, Meyer, Kung & Sullivan, in press). Assigning students within the same school to treatment conditions is more likely to result in similar groups across treatment conditions. Students within the same school come from the same neighborhoods and are more likely to be similar than students from different schools. In contrast, differences in school size, teachers, school atmosphere, school policies, and the presence of other ongoing programs can complicate the interpretation of between-school designs. Such differences make it difficult to determine the extent to which schools differ because of their participation in RIPP or because of other differences that have nothing to do with RIPP. Within-school designs also make it possible to offer the program to at least some of the students at each participating school. This can avoid some of the morale problems encountered when schools that are not directly benefiting from the program are asked to provide data and cooperate with other aspects of the evaluation.

A significant advantage of between-school designs is that they avoid potential problems with diffusion effects (Kazdin, 1998). Diffusion of treatment occurs when students not assigned to the intervention are exposed to some of its elements through their interactions with peers, teachers, and others who participate in the intervention. Interventions can have a variety of indirect effects on nonparticipants. For example, students who participate in an intervention may be less likely to become involved in fights on the school playground not only with each other, but with nonparticipants as well. Piecemeal implementation of an intervention within a school may also not provide the same benefits as schoolwide implementation. For example, it may not be possible to evaluate components such as peer mediation, teacher training, and other strategies designed to produce overall changes in school environment (e.g., changes in school policies). Finally, the choice of a between-school or within-school design will often be based on practical considerations. Assignment of entire schools to treatment conditions can be attempted only when there is a sufficient number of schools to assign several schools to each condition. Such designs may not be feasible in small school systems or when individuals at a single school are interested in implementing RIPP.

Regardless of whether schools, classrooms, or individual students are assigned to treatment conditions, it is essential that some method of random assignment be used. There is a natural tendency to allocate resources where they are most needed. If left unchecked, this can cause decision-makers to assign schools, classes, or students that have the greatest need to the intervention group. The flip side of this is that schools, classes, or students that have the least need are assigned to the control group by default, and they do not provide an adequate comparison group for evaluating the impact of the program. Random assignment (e.g., drawing names out of a hat) is a preferred method because it means that every school or student has an equal chance of being in each of the treatment conditions. This strategy is more likely to result in groups that are equivalent before they participate in the intervention. Such equivalence makes it easier to attribute any observed differences to the effects of intervention.

Random assignment does not always result in equivalent groups. For example, suppose that four of the ten schools in a particular school system serve a high percentage of students who live in low-income housing projects. Random assignment of these schools could result in three or four of these schools being assigned to the same treatment condition. One method of addressing this problem is to match schools or groups of students before random assignment. In the current example, each of the ten schools could be paired with whichever school was most similar. Within each of these ten pairs of schools, one would be randomly assigned to each of the two treatment conditions. Such an approach can be an effective in reducing differences between schools or students assigned to each treatment condition.

MEASURING PROGRAM IMPACT

Conducting an evaluation of RIPP also involves the selecting measures designed to assess the impact of the program. This process begins by identifying the short-term and long-term objectives of the program (e.g., see Figure 4.1). The extent to which each objective is accomplished must be assessed by collecting data on a measure that accurately reflects each objective. For example, if a school system's primary reason for implementing RIPP is to reduce fights on school grounds, it would obviously be important to include a measure of this behavior.

Evaluators should be realistic about their program objectives and avoid including measures that are unlikely to be influenced by the intervention. For example, although reducing adolescents' exposure to violence in their community might be a very desirable outcome, it is unlikely that a school-based program could produce such a change. Measures should also be sensitive to treatment changes. For example, a measure that includes questions such as whether students have ever been in trouble with the police or court system may be of limited value. If the students were in trouble with the courts before participating in the intervention, their answers will not change after they complete the intervention. It is therefore better to include questions that relate to a shorter period of time (e.g., the last 30 days).

The selection of appropriate measures should also be guided by the characteristics of the students who participate in the evaluation. Measures should be age-appropriate for use with middle school students. Other student characteristics and setting variables should also be considered. For example, we constructed a scale to assess students' reactions to hypothetical problem situations that included situations identified by students within our urban, predominantly African-American student population (Farrell, Ampy, & Meyer, 1998). Contextual factors can also be very important in interpreting the meaning of items. In our evaluation of the RIPP program in the rural schools, we were initially shocked by the high percentage of students who reported that they had "heard guns being shot" and "carried a weapon." We felt rather foolish when it was later explained to that these students live in areas where hunting is common. These items carried a rather different interpretation in the urban setting where they were originally used.

Efforts should also be made to include multiple sources of data. Our evaluations of RIPP have typically included both student reports and data based on disciplinary code violations. Although self-report measures are often criticized for being too subjective and susceptible to bias (e.g., students trying to make themselves look good), others have argued that, under proper circumstances, adolescents tend to be reasonably truthful in reporting problem behaviors. Indeed, such data form the basis of national studies of trends in behaviors such as drug use among adolescents (e.g., Johnston, 1985; Oetting & Beauvais, 1990). The accuracy of a self-report clearly depends upon the conditions in which it is obtained. In our evaluations of RIPP, we attempt to create an environment in which students are comfortable giving honest responses. Where possible, we employ staff that are not associated with the school system, so that school officials are not involved in handling data. These staff members are trained to address student concerns regarding confidentiality. Student names do not appear on any of the test materials, and we employ statistical criteria to screen out random responders (Farrell, Danish, & Howard, 1991).

Each assessment method has its own inherent problems. In presentations of our evaluation findings, we have found that audiences tend to be the most impressed with changes we report on school disciplinary code violations (e.g., suspensions for fighting). These are generally regarded as more objective than student reports. These data are not, however, without their own interpretation problems. Disciplinary code violations underestimate occurrences of problem behaviors because not all fights or other incidents occur on school grounds, students are not always caught, and disciplinary rules are not always consistently enforced. Other sources of data obtained from collateral sources such as parents and teachers may also be difficult to interpret because they are unlikely to witness all incidents of problem behavior. Because there is no incontrovertible method of measuring problem behavior that can be used in all situations, multiple sources should be used whenever possible.

School systems that conduct evaluations of RIPP can refer to several sources that may help guide the selection of instruments. Table 4.1 provides a list of some of the measures of key objectives that we have used in our own evaluations of the RIPP program. Additional details regarding these measures may be found in previous studies we have published (Farrell, Kung, White, & Valois, in press; Farrell & Meyer, 1997) or on our project web site www.has.vcu.edu/RIPP. Although this may provide a useful starting point, evaluations in other school systems should employ measures that best represent their project objectives and characteristics of the students in their school system. A useful source for such measures is a compendium of measures published by the Centers for Disease Control and Prevention (CDC) (Dahlberg, Toal, & Behrens, 1998). This document lists more than 100 measures used by 15 CDC-funded projects that evaluated violence prevention programs. It includes measures of attitudes and beliefs related to aggression, psychosocial and cognitive variables (e.g., attributional bias, ethnic identity, moral reasoning), behavior (e.g., conflict resolution skills, parental control, leisure activity), and environment (e.g., family environment, quality of neighborhood).

TIMING OF DATA COLLECTION

Developing an appropriate evaluative design requires selecting of appropriate measures of program effects and also determining the most appropriate times to collect these data. At a minimum, program evaluations provide for collecting of data at pretest and post-test. Pretest data, which are collected before to implementing any aspect of the program, provide a starting point for assessing change. They also provide an opportunity to determine if the students assigned to different treatment conditions are equivalent. It is difficult to interpret differences in pre-to-post changes across groups if the groups are not the same to begin with.

The timing of post-test data is also important. These data should be collected after the intervention has been completed, should reflect an appropriate window of time, and should provide sufficient time for program effects to occur. The importance of waiting until the program has been completed before collect-

Table 4.1. Examples of Measures Used to Evaluate RIPP

Objective	Measure	Description
	Proximal Program Objectives	
To increase knowledge of the material covered in the curriculum	RIPP Knowledge Test	An 18-item multiple choice test covering knowledge of RIPP principles. The total score reflects the number of correct answers.
To create favorable attitudes toward nonviolent methods of addressing problems	Attitudes Toward Violence and Nonviolence Scales	Students indicate the extent to which they agree or disagree with 13 items reflecting attitudes that favor violent and nonviolent behaviors. Separate scales reflect their opinions of using violent and nonviolent behaviors.
To increase peer support for nonviolent methods of addressing problems	Peer Support for Nonviolence Scale	Students indicate how they think their friends would react if they responded to hypothetical problem situations with various violent and nonviolent strategies. Total score represents the degree of perceived support for choosing nonviolent reactions.
To increase the use of nonviolent methods for addressing conflict	Problem Situation Inventory	Students select the response that best represents what they would do in six different hypothetical conflict situations. The total score reflects the number of times they chose a nonviolent strategy.
To increase impulse control	Weinberger Adjustment Inventory Impulse Control Subscale	An 8-item scale that assesses the student's tendency to act in impulsive ways.
	Distal Program Objectives	
To reduce the frequency of aggression	Behavioral Frequency Scales—Aggression Subscale	Students report how frequently they engaged in 14 behaviors representing various acts of physical and nonphysical aggression in the past 30 days.
	Interpersonal Problem Situations for Urban Adolescents—Peer Provocation Subscale	Students indicate how frequently they were exposed to specific examples of peer provocation in the past 30 days.
	School Disciplinary Code Violations	The frequency of school disciplinary code violations related to violent behaviors, as reported by the school.

ing post-test data is apparent. Although participants may begin to show some changes while participating in RIPP, the full benefits of the program will not be observed until they have completed it. It is not enough that post-test data be collected after completing of treatment, the time frame it represents should also not overlap participation in treatment. Practical constraints imposed by the school calendar may make this latter requirement difficult to satisfy. In our own evaluations of RIPP-6, we have examined, the effects of intervention by noting changes in disciplinary code violations for the last quarter of the 6th-grade school year and changes in measures completed by students at the end of the school year that assess their frequency of engaging in problem behaviors during the preceding 30 days. Because the 25-session RIPP-6 program is typically completed near the end of the school year, the time frame for both of these types of measures commences before the program has been completed.

A further complication with obtaining measures of program effects immediately after participants have completed the program is that it may not allow sufficient time for program effects to emerge. In some cases, a program may even produce negative effects at post-test. For example, in several evaluations of RIPP-6, we have noted that participants sometimes show increases in the frequency of fighting on post-test measures (Farrell, Meyer, Kung & Sullivan, in press). These findings suggest that participants in the intervention may initially have limited success applying the new skills they learned. They may even be less successful avoiding fights than before the intervention. The acquisition of new skills may take time, and students may not use these skills until they feel they have successfully mastered them or have an opportunity to apply them in new settings. Therefore, evaluations conducted on post-test data collected immediately after completing of the program must be interpreted very cautiously.

Collection of follow-up data can provide an effective means of addressing some of the previously noted problems with post-test data and can provide a basis for determining the extent to which program effects are maintained over time. Our evaluations of RIPP-6 have included follow-up assessments completed 6 months and 12 months after students completed the program. Analyses of these data have been extremely valuable. The findings at our 6-month follow-up indicated that the initial increase in physical fighting among RIPP participants noted immediately after completing of the program reversed itself. We also found that some of the positive benefits of the program were maintained at the 6-month assessment, and significant effects emerged on several other variables (e.g., threatening teachers, skipping school because of concerns about safety) that had not been evident at the post-test. The findings of our 12-month follow-up of RIPP-6 have also been useful. In general, we found that the positive effects observed earlier were no longer evident a year after completing of the program. These findings led to the development of the RIPP-7 and RIPP-8 curricula that were designed to strengthen and extend the RIPP-6 curriculum.

Although follow-up assessments can provide important information about long-term program effects, they should be interpreted cautiously because of the selective effects of attrition. With the passage of time, it may become increasingly difficult to collect data from all of the students who participated in an evaluation.

Students move, transfer to other schools, are expelled, are not promoted, are absent on the day measures are administered, or elect not to participate in the evaluation. A negative consequence is that the resulting sample of students may no longer adequately represent those who initially participated in the evaluation. This is supported by the results of our evaluations that have found that students for whom follow-up data are not available tend to be those who reported higher rates of problem behaviors on earlier assessments (Farrell & Meyer, 1997; Farrell et al., 1999). Their absence at follow-up assessments can mask effects. For example, our evaluation of RIPP-6 (Farrell et al., 1999) found that significant pre-to-post program effects on disciplinary code violations for carrying weapons and for fight-related injuries were no longer significant at the 6-month follow-up. Further examination of the data revealed that many of the students who had disciplinary code violations for fighting and carrying weapons at the post-test assessment did not return to the same school for the 7th grade. The net effect was that students in the control group who were more likely to have had problems were also more likely to be excluded from the 6-month follow-up.

CONCLUSIONS

Conducting a well-designed evaluation of a prevention program such as RIPP can be a daunting task that may require considerable resources. Such evaluations, however, are well worth the cost and effort involved. The process of implementing a program such as RIPP also requires resources, and the continued implementation of such a program without evidence that it is achieving its desired effects is not likely to be cost-effective in the long run. Beyond determining if a program is working, evaluation findings can also be of considerable value in improving a program's effectiveness. This is a basic element of the action-research strategy we employed in developing RIPP. Others interested in addressing a significant social problem such as youth violence are encouraged to continue this process by integrating evaluation into their plans for implementing RIPP or other prevention programs directed at addressing such problems.

There is no shortage of violence prevention programs designed for use in school settings. There is, however, a shortage of data that can help decision-makers identify the most effective program to use with a given population in a particular type of setting. This situation will not improve without some effort to determine the effectiveness of these programs. Readers interested in implementing RIPP within their schools may find themselves overwhelmed by the prospect of conducting a large scale evaluation project. Such readers should not be discouraged. The types of comprehensive designs described in this chapter represent end points of a project. Such end points may emerge from more humble beginnings. Our own efforts to develop an effective program to address youth violence began with very simplistic designs. We did not have the resources or commitment from the community to implement more rigorous evaluations until several years into the project. We also learned the value of piloting interventions before they are evaluated. This approach will not quickly lead to progress but will provide a foundation for such progress. As Mercy and Potter noted: "The problem of violence in America did not appear overnight, nor will it disappear suddenly. A sustained and coordinated effort to prevent violence will be necessary at all levels of society to address this complex and deeply rooted problem" (1996, p. 2).

What Works:

- Comprehensive strategies designed to evaluate the process of program implementation and program impact on immediate and longer term objectives (see Figure 4.1). Ideally, such designs should involve multiple schools, should obtain data from multiple sources, and should provide for collecting long-term follow-up data.
- The inclusion of a process evaluation to indicate the extent to which the program was faithfully implemented and to identify variables that may have influenced the program's effectiveness.
- The evaluation of a program's impact on immediate objectives to provide a basis for determining if participants are getting the immediate benefits expected from the program and to identify adjustments that may be needed in program content or implementation if they are not.
- Evaluations of a program's impact on longer term objectives to provide a basis for determining the extent to which the program is achieving its ultimate objectives.
- Combining all three strategies within the context of an action-research model to provide a basis for continually refining a program, identifying the necessary conditions for it to be successful, and identifying those students who are most likely to benefit.

What Doesn't Work:

- The continued practice of devoting resources to implementing of programs of unproven effectiveness. Such an effort may lead decision-makers into believing that they are doing something to address the problem of youth violence, when little is actually being accomplished.
- The implementation of poorly designed evaluations. Some information is not better than no information if the information is not accurate. There is little to be gained by conducting ill-designed evaluations and much to be lost.

What Might Work:

- Efforts to evaluate RIPP implemented on a small scale within a single school. During the early stage of this process, the emphasis should be on process evaluation. Efforts should be made to overcome obstacles to program implementation, to document that the program is being implemented as it was designed, to clarify modifications made to accommodate local circumstances related to the setting or student population, and to identify which students are being served.
- The use of more comprehensive designs in subsequent years. The impact of the program can be evaluated by conducting a within-school design, perhaps using data that are already routinely collected (e.g., school disciplinary code violations, visits to the nurses office for fight-related injuries). Then, these data may provide the basis for obtaining the funding and resources needed to conduct more rigorous evaluations. Such an effort may lead to the pooling of resources across schools or school systems.

5

Overview of RIPP-6

This chapter provides an overview of RIPP-6, the 25-session violence prevention curriculum designed for the first year of either middle school (6th grade) or junior high school (7th grade). After the essence and core components of RIPP are described, a description of the manual and the strategies used in the program are presented. A short summary of the goals for each session is provided, followed by a sample workshop. The standardized RIPP-6 instructor manual (approximately 200 pages) is available through the RIPP Project Office and is intended to be used in tandem with the guidance in operations and evaluation that is provided in this monograph.

THE ESSENCE OF RIPP-6

The RIPP-6 program is designed to let students know that they have choices when they find themselves in conflict situations. Moving to middle or junior high school is a very difficult transition for many students. For example, school expectations change, and the content of classes gets harder; puberty (or the expectation of puberty) stimulates new and sometimes confusing feelings; and although early adolescents still feel very attached to their parents, they are developing more intense relationships with their peers. All too many students in middle or junior high school, after getting into a fight, will act as if the violence was inevitable because "he got in my space" or "she told a lie about me." They instinctively believe in the "fight or flight" theory: you can either wimp out and walk away, or you can stay and fight it out, thus saving face and winning.

Moreover, we have learned that many fights are motivated by the need to resolve a conflict, and also because fighting can provide desired outcomes for those involved. For example, students frequently report that there are more positive consequences to getting into a fight (e.g., gaining status, relieving steam, proving your point) than negative consequences (e.g., getting caught). Unfortunately, some programs designed for this age group teach a form of conflict resolution that focuses solely on talking out a problem, ignoring other options, as well as the fact that fighting can be a road to goal attainment for some students. In RIPP-6, we focus on helping youth see that they have a *variety* of choices as they face conflict, that choosing a nonviolent alternative has desirable consequences, and that nonviolent alternatives work well in the real world.

In summary, the motto of RIPP is embedded in the idea of personal responsibility in the face of choices → You can Respond In Peaceful and Positive Ways, or you can Rest In Peace Permanently, the choice is YOURS!! The core problem-solving model for RIPP is represented by the acronym SCIDDLE, and the core skills are represented by the acronym RAID (see Figure 5.1). Ideally, the RIPP-6 classroom provides an opportunity for students to explore non-violent options for conflict resolution and achievement that they might otherwise not have the opportunity to experience directly.

Standardized Curriculum Manual

Each of the 25 sessions in the standardized RIPP curriculum manual begins with a page that describes the session's goals, key points, and necessary materials and preparation. The specified activities, estimated time required for each activity, detailed directions, sample lectures, and instructional resource pages are provided for each session. These details are provided to optimize the consistency of the program across instructors. Basic social learning principles (Bandura, 1986) are used for instructing each session, whereby the prevention facilitators (1) name and describe what is being taught, (2) facilitate discussion as to why the material and/or skill is of value, (3) provide models that demonstrate the particular topic, and (4) facilitate skill practice and provide feedback as appropriate.

Stop.
Calm down.
Identify the problem and your feelings about it.
Decide among your options → Resolve, Avoid, Ignore, Diffuse
Do it!
Look back.
Evaluate.

Figure 5.1. SCIDDLE problem-solving model and RAID skills.

EDUCATIONAL STRATEGIES AND CONTENT

The very structure of the lessons and the tone of the classroom help model a positive approach to conflict resolution. Whereas the facilitator is clearly in control in the classroom, he or she participates in all the activities and truly *facilitates* the discussion, thus sharing the power of having the "right" answer. Many young people at this age feel very powerless, and they experience many of the adults they encounter using power in inappropriate ways. The facilitation process demonstrates a different view of power.

Building group cohesion is crucial to the success of the RIPP program because students will need to develop a certain sense of safety and trust with this particular group of peers if they are to try alternatives to violent behavior in role-plays and discussions. Most of the activities in beginning sessions are designed to build group cohesion; they are opportunities for the students to get to know each other a little better in a safe, nonthreatening way. They will have a chance to laugh with each other, and this is an important community builder. Unlike some other academic subjects, students will not be able to learn the concepts in RIPP unless there is peer acceptance for learning these concepts. Spending time in the beginning and throughout the program building and enhancing this peer acceptance is quite important.

A combination of three basic strategies is used throughout the curriculum: behavioral repetition and mental rehearsal of a social-cognitive problem-solving model, experiential learning techniques, and guided discussions. The problem-solving model provides the backbone for the entire curriculum; each session builds upon the previous ones, using the entire model cumulatively. The early sessions focus on team-building and knowledge transmission (Sessions 1–11), and the later sessions focus on skill-building (Sessions 12–17, 19, 21, and 23) and critical analysis (Sessions 18, 20, 22, 24–25).

The Social-Cognitive Problem-Solving Model. The seven-step social-cognitive problem-solving model is represented by the acronym **SCIDDLE** (Meyer & Northup, 1998): **S**top; **C**alm down; **I**dentify the problem and your feelings about it; **D**ecide among your options; **D**o it; **L**ook back; and **E**valuate. This model emphasizes the importance of calming down, choosing among prosocial options, and looking back to determine if the course of action taken was in line with one's own values and priorities.

The four prosocial options provided for preventing violence within this model are *Resolve, Avoid, Ignore,* and *Diffuse* (represented by the acronym **RAID**). By teaching these four skills, the RIPP program makes explicit the need for adolescents to think ahead about all types of situations that might lead to violence and to consider options for preventing that violence. For example, a conflict related to teasing between two girls could be addressed through any of these four strategies, depending upon the details of the situation. For two girls who are close friends, using *resolve* (e.g., talking through the problem or going to peer mediation) would be an appropriate response. In contrast, if they are not friends and have a history of fighting, talking through the problem alone might not be appropriate (although going to peer mediation might be). Instead, if the two girls were to *avoid* each other, this could help prevent the problem in the first place. If such a solution is not possible, using *ignore* might be effective, especially if each uses positive self-talk statements (e.g., "She's just having a bad day" or "I know I am a good person no matter what others say about me"). *Diffuse*, a more complex strategy that calls for decreasing the amount of tension in the situation, might be effective if either girl (1) tried to imagine what it felt like to be in the other's shoes, (2) apologized, or (3) realized that she did not have to "expect the worst" or "take the bait." Because the curriculum emphasizes frequent use of role-plays with group discussions of multiple prosocial responses to potential conflicts, we expect that students will learn to make effective choices about which strategy to use, given the situation and his/her personal abilities (i.e., Objective 12).

Experiential Learning Strategies. A wide range of experiential learning strategies is used to optimize participation by all members of the class. These strategies include trust-building activities, relaxation techniques, small group work, role-playing, journal writing, and reflection on these activities. The use of small groups in which students work together to achieve a common goal and to participate in various roles (i.e., leader, reporter, recorder), is particularly important in RIPP. This promotes cooperation, increases awareness of the value of each individual to the larger group, and helps diminish stereotypes that students might have about themselves and others.

Guided Discussions. Guided discussions following mini-lectures, videos, and questionnaires are used periodically throughout the curriculum to increase students' knowledge about the nature of violence and nonviolence. For example, in Session 4, "Making RIPP Real," the prevention facilitator introduces four story lines about conflict that will be followed throughout the year. Each of the four story lines focuses on recent news in one of these four areas: local news, national news, sports, and celebrities. The use of story lines from recent news items helps make the program material come to life for the students and demonstrates the facilitator's awareness of important community events. It is our contention that information about violence can be used to promote motivation within the students to learn skills that promote a positive and peaceful society.

THE 25 SESSIONS OF RIPP-6

As described in Chapter 1, RIPP-6 consists of 25 fifty-minute sessions that are to be taught once a week for 25 weeks. Below is a short description of the goals for each session.

Session 1: Getting Acquainted

The goals for this workshop are to get acquainted with the students and to introduce the concept of choice in RIPP.

Session 2: Impact

The goal of this workshop is to increase the students' awareness of the impact that violence can have on the quality of life.

Session 3: Ground Rules and Introduction to SCIDDLE and RAID

The goals of this session are for the students to get to know each other better, to talk about the facts related to homicide, to establish ground rules, and to introduce the RIPP problem-solving model (SCIDDLE and RAID).

Session 4: Making RIPP Real

The goals of this session are to familiarize students with each step of the RIPP problem-solving model, to discuss the positive and negative aspects of conflict, and to select "story lines" about conflict that can be followed throughout the year to "Make RIPP Real."

Session 5: Stop and Calm Down

The goals of this session are to teach students about the relationship between physiology and emotion, to teach them to identify their own physical signals of anger and anxiety, and to introduce various healthy ways to calm down. The breathing technique taught in this lesson can be used at the beginning of each session to help the students focus on RIPP.

Session 6: Identifying Your Feelings

The primary goal of this session is to provide an opportunity for the students to role-play feelings, to become familiar with the different types of emotions; and to identify cues that indicate one's own and others' feelings. This is the first workshop that focuses on the "I" step of SCIDDLE: Identifying the problem and your feelings about it.

Session 7: Identifying the Problem I: Group Survival

The primary goals of this class are to teach the students to work in small groups. Although role-playing may be the obvious time when students are learning communication skills in RIPP, learning to work in small groups is just as important for practicing the same skills.

Session 8: Identifying the Problem II: Differences

The goals of this lesson are to explain how differences are often the cause of conflicts, to teach that differences can be constructive, and to provide students with opportunities to recognize and affirm differences.

Session 9: Identifying the Problem III: Diversity and the American Dream

The goals of this lesson are for everyone to explore his or her own cultural heritage, to learn about the heritage of others, to consider how these differences influence the "American Dream," and to think about what the "American Dream" might mean to them in the future.

Session 10: Identifying the Problem IV: The Violence Web

The goal of this lesson is to demonstrate to students that violence feeds upon itself to create more and more violence.

Session 11: Identifying Solutions: The RIPP Web of Support

The goals of this session are to demonstrate ways in which RAID can be used to block violence, to create an alternative to the Violence Web (the RIPP Web of Support), and to emphasize that each person is personally responsible for making deliberate choices about which type of community he/she wants to promote.

Session 12: Decide Option One: Avoid

This session marks the beginning of a number of skill-building workshops. The primary goal of this lesson is to help the students understand the strategy of *avoid* as an option for violence prevention and the times when it would be most appropriate. The secondary goal is to teach the students about nonverbal behavior as it relates to violence and aggression.

Session 13: Decide Option Two: Ignore

The primary goal of this lesson is to help the students understand the strategy of *ignore* as an option for violence prevention and the times when this strategy would be most appropriate. The secondary goal is to teach students the value of using self-talk to figure out how to deal with problems.

Session 14: Decide Option Three: When to Diffuse

The goal of this session is to get the students to think about how "expecting the worst" and "taking the bait" (i.e., negative attributions) set a person up to get into a fight. The concept of *diffuse* will be introduced.

Session 15: Decide Option Three: How to Diffuse

The goal of this workshop is to expose the students to a wide range of techniques for diffusing a conflict situation, as well as to provide opportunities to role-play those techniques.

Session 16: Decide Option Four: Resolving by Fighting Fair

The goal of this workshop is to expose the students to examples of *resolve* techniques as well as to provide opportunities for discussion of the Civil Rights movement.

Session 17: Doing it One: Role-Playing Resolve

The goal of this workshop is to get the students to role-play using the fighting fair rules to resolve a problem situation.

Session 18: Look Back and Evaluate One: Who is Responsible

The goal of this session is to begin focusing on the last two steps of SCIDDLE (Look back and Evaluate) by considering what people and factors were responsible for the problem. The students will be challenged to think about the future roles they will have as adults (worker, family member, and citizen) and how carrying them out responsibly helps the whole community. Their current roles as student and community member as bystanders will be examined.

Session 19: Doing It Two: Peer Mediation

The goal of this session is to educate and familiarize the students with peer mediation (as part of the *resolve* option of RAID). There will be opportunities to think about how peer mediation is an example of being a responsible friend, citizen, and family member.

Session 20: Look Back and Evaluate II: Values

The purpose of this workshop is to continue focusing on the last part of SCIDDLE. It will introduce students to the concept of values and encourage them to explore their own values (especially about violence). They will also be given a homework activity to help them think about the influence of media on their values.

Session 21: Doing It Three: Ways to Resolve in the Family

The goals of this workshop are to get the students to explore what they think of families, how they would like their future family to be, and to discuss why parents have some of the rules that they do.

Session 22: Look Back and Evaluate III: Critical Consumers of Violent Media

This lesson is designed to help the students understand the effect that violence in the media has on them and to raise their ability to consume this material critically by comparing the messages across many types of media. A particular focus of this workshop is to examine what types of negative images media perpetuate about each gender.

Session 23: Doing It Four: Role-Playing SCIDDLE

The purpose of this session is to provide an opportunity for students to apply the entire SCIDDLE problem-solving model to different situations.

Session 24: Making a Pledge of Nonviolence

The goal of this concluding session is to affirm students for the hard work they have done during the year and for the decisions that they will make as a result of that work. We also hope that one decision students will make is to sign a pledge to use constructive means (i.e., SCIDDLE and RAID) to solve their conflicts in the future.

Session 25: World Party

The goal of the final session is to celebrate the completion of RIPP-6 with poster-making and a party.

SAMPLE SESSION

SESSION 8—Identifying the Problem II: DIFFERENCES

Goal

The goals of this lesson are to explain how differences are often the cause of conflicts, to teach that differences can be constructive, and to provide students with opportunities to recognize and affirm differences.

Key Concepts

- DIFFERENCES: Everyone is both similar and different from other people. The world would be a boring place if everyone were alike. It is important to recognize that although differences are positive, they can be a source of conflict.
- STEREOTYPE: The belief that all people in a certain group are alike. Stereotypes do not allow for individuality; they are images that may become frozen in our minds.
- TOLERANCE: Recognizing and respecting the differences of those different from ourselves.

Materials and Preparation Checklist

- Newsprint or wipe-off board
- Markers
- Masking tape
- Cut up cereal boxes (14 pieces)
- Review questions handout
- Two bandanas

CLASSROOM ACTIVITIES

I. Review and Introduction (2 minutes)

Ask the students to name all of the different roles that there are in small groups. Ask them what they have done so far to learn how to use SCIDDLE. Explain that today they will be learning more about the I-step (Identify the Problem) and about the way differences are sometimes the source of problems. Ask the students the following question:

"How many of you don't have a problem with people who are different?"

Count how many raise their hands (probably very few will). Refer to this question later on when students are gaining more awareness of their own stereotypes and prejudices.

Remember, you may want to start the sessions with practice of the breathing technique for calming down.

II. Tolerance (15 minutes)

This activity is designed to demonstrate physical differences, as well as to show how people can work together for a common task. Ask for four volunteers. Explain that they have been on a space mission to a planet that has very little water. The spacecraft crashed on the planet. The crew survived; however, two lost their sight, and the other two lost the use of their arms. All that is left from the spacecraft is one radio transmitter, one weather machine, pieces of the spacecraft, and some tape. The weather machine just indicated that it is going to rain in four minutes and the crew needs to get the water to survive until the rescue team arrives. Tell the volunteers that they will have four minutes to make containers that will catch the rain.

Pair them up. In each pair, blindfold one volunteer and have the other volunteer hold her/his hands behind her/his back. Give each pair seven pieces of the spacecraft (cut up cereal boxes) and one long piece of masking tape. Coach each group to stay on task, directing them to take some deep breaths if they need to calm down. After four minutes, remove the blindfolds, and have each pair present their container to the large group.

Ask questions such as the following:

1. *What was different in this situation?*
2. *What was it like to be blindfolded? not to be able to use your hands?*
3. *What was the lesson?*
4. *Is it true that we all have strengths and weaknesses?*
5. *Would you continue to be friends with someone if they lost their sight?*

6. *How do you treat people with mental handicaps?*
7. *What is a stereotype? Define.*
8. *How many of you still think you don't have a problem with people who are different from you?*

III. Face to Face (15 minutes)

The purpose of this activity is to highlight how everyone is similar to and different from everyone else. Determine the number of students. Divide that number in half and have the students count off. Students with the same numbers make a pair.

Explain the activity as follows:

Now we are going to find out how we are alike and how we are different. I want you to find out five things in which you and your partner are the same and five that are different. Remember what these ten things are, as I will be asking you to remember afterwards. You have 5 minutes.

Wander around the room to be sure the pairs are staying on target. When the five minutes are up, ask the students for examples of similarities and differences.

Point out how many similarities and differences there were in the answers the students gave. Point out that they can choose whether these differences become problems or these differences make their school a more interesting place to be.

IV. Closure and Review Questions (5 minutes)

Thank the students for exploring ways in which they are different and similar to others in their classroom. Explain that in the next session they will be exploring their cultural heritage. Direct students to find out where their names come from and what they mean by asking their parents, grandparents, or relatives.

Review sessions 5–8 with the students. Hand out review questions, review them, and return them to your supervisor.

Instructional Resource Page for Session 8

Experiential Learning and Reflection. One of the key elements of experiential learning is reflection on the activity. This is when students have an opportunity to think about what they just did and what it meant to them at the moment. Then, they can begin to abstract that experience and apply it to past and potential future experiences. It is important in experiential learning for students to arrive at the learning through this reflection; the facilitator should not tell them what they should have learned. However, asking probing questions can sometimes guide students to insights they might not otherwise have had. For example, with the "Tolerance" activity, probing questions can help the volunteers articulate their feelings about being handicapped (i.e., blind-folded or hands tied) and then use their experience to increase their understanding of people who are different from them.

Name _____

RIPP REVIEW (5-8)

The questions below review the different things that were taught in RIPP. Please read each question, think about your answer, and then write your answer. Your honest answer will help us to improve the program.

1. Why is it important to stop and calm down before you act?

2. What are three things you can do to <u>stop and calm down</u>?

3. What is one good thing about differences?

4. What is one bad thing about differences?

6

Overview of RIPP-7

This chapter provides an overview of RIPP-7, the 12-session violence prevention curriculum designed for the second year of either middle school (7th grade) or junior high school (8th grade). Once the essence and core components of RIPP-7 are described, a description of the strategies used in the program is presented. A short summary of the goals for each session is provided, as well as a sample workshop. The standardized RIPP-7 instructor manual (approximately 100 pages) is available through the Life Skills Center and is intended to be used in tandem with the guidance in operations and evaluation that is provided in this monograph.

THE ESSENCE OF RIPP-7

The focus of the second year of RIPP is on teaching the more complex skill of conflict resolution (i.e., resolve). Our experience has shown us that we can capitalize on the increasing social maturity of youth to demonstrate the value of conflict resolution as an important part of friendship. We expect that friendship is a context where students can safely experiment with conflict resolution. As they resolve conflicts with their friends, they will learn one of the key benefits of this skill → Working through conflict makes things even better! Once students have mastered conflict resolution in the domain of friendship, they can attempt transferring the skill to other relationships in their lives. Ideally, as students learn to use conflict resolution successfully, they will continue to learn the benefits of nonviolence, thus reducing their need and/or desire to engage in violent behavior.

The acronym that represents the skills learned in RIPP-7 is RSLV (See Figure 6.1). This acronym is a play on the skill *resolve* and includes the important steps of listening to others and communicating clearly. This acronym also in-

Respect Others → Listen to what they have to say!

Speak Clearly → How else can they understand what you mean?!

Listen to Yourself → What you want is important!

Value the Friendship → Isn't that what life is all about?!

Figure 6.1. RSLV Conflict Resolution Skills for Friendship.

cludes the skill *diffuse*. For example, one of the most powerful ways to *diffuse* a conflict is to respect the person with whom you are in conflict; another effective way to diffuse is to stay centered by listening to yourself and remembering what is most important to you.

EDUCATIONAL STRATEGIES AND CONTENT

Although the teaching strategies in RIPP-7 are the same as those in RIPP-6, one significant difference is the increased use of experiential activities to demonstrate concepts taught in the curriculum. In particular, activities modified from the martial art of Aikido (Crum, 1987) are used to provide physical and personal examples of the way various conflict resolution skills work. Much of the philosophy of Aikido is expressed in the following idea: "Identify with the enemy and they are transformed" (Galland, 1980).

THE 12 SESSIONS OF RIPP-7

As described in Chapter 1, RIPP-7 consists of 12 fifty-minute sessions designed to be taught weekly. Following is a short description of the goals for each session.

Session 1: Introduction and Review

The primary goals of this session are for the facilitator to introduce himself/herself, to develop a set of ground rules with each class, and to get to know the students.

Session 2: Making RIPP Real Again

The goals of this session are to illustrate the relationships between change, stress, and conflict and to "make this real" by showing how each of these sometimes lead to acquaintance and interpersonal violence.

Session 3: Respect

The goals of this class are to get the students thinking about respect and disrespect, to review and practice working in small groups, to demonstrate how one way of showing respect is to acknowledge another person's role, and to demonstrate how following our own values is one way we show respect to ourselves.

Session 4: Friendship and Conflict

The primary goals of this class are to discuss friendship, to consider how conflict works in friendships, and to learn more about one of the most important skills for friendship—being a good listener.

Session 5: Using RSLV in Relationships

The goals of this session are to explain RSLV and to show how resolving issues can help to reduce conflicts in friendships.

Session 6: Calm Down and Listen to Yourself

The primary goal of this session is to reinforce the value of calming yourself down physiologically before responding to a problem situation. The secondary goal is to introduce the idea that when we are calm, it is easier to listen to ourselves and do what we really want. Short-term and long-term techniques for calming down will be presented.

Session 7: Listening to Others

The goals of this workshop are to increase students' awareness of the value of listening and to teach them skills for listening.

Session 8: Speaking So Others Can Listen

The goals of this session are to encourage the students to try using nonconfrontational language in resolving conflicts and to get them to take responsibility for their own feelings in a conflict.

Session 9: Asking Yourself "What Do I Want?"

The goal of this lesson is to help students decide what outcome they want to achieve from an interaction and to choose methods for achieving that goal appropriately.

Session 10: Putting RSLV Together I

In this session, students have the opportunity to develop role-plays using the skills for RSLV.

Session 11: Putting RSLV Together II

This session builds on the previous one by giving students the opportunity to share their role-plays with the rest of the class.

Session 12: Closure and Commitment

The goals of the closing workshop are to emphasize how much the students have learned about preventing acquaintance violence by reviewing RSLV, making a group commitment for nonviolence, and making individual pledges for nonviolence.

SAMPLE SESSION

Session 4: Friendships and Conflict

Goal

The primary goals of this class are to discuss friendship, to consider how conflict works in friendships, and to learn more about one of the most important skills for friendship—being a good listener.

Key Concepts

- *Liking yourself:* Before someone can like you, you have to like yourself.
- *Making friends:* The best way to make a friend is by being a friend.
- *Conflict:* A struggle or clashing between views and opinions.

Materials and Preparation Checklist

- Newsprint or wipe-off board, index cards, and markers
- Small group worksheet on Conflicts in Friendships
- Practice the Tenkan game with a friend

CLASSROOM ACTIVITIES

I. Review and Introduction (7 min.)

Review the concepts of respect and disrespect by applying them to friendship. Say to the students:

> The last time we were together we talked a lot about respect and disrespect. As a way of reviewing those two concepts and applying them to an area of life that is important for 7th graders, let's make two lists. One list is things 7th graders say, do, and think that show respect to their friends. The other list is things 7th graders say, do, and think that show disrespect to their friends.

Make two columns on the board and write in the students' ideas. After the students have offered many ideas, begin a discussion of conflict in friendship by asking the students:

1. If someone has a friend, why would that person do any of these things that show disrespect?
2. What happens to a friendship if we do lots of disrespectful things to the other person?
3. Do people sometimes show disrespect when they are having a conflict in a friendship?
4. Sometimes when a friend disrespects us, but we ignore it, that is an example of us not respecting ourselves—of disrespecting ourselves. When we do this, it is a sign that we do not like ourselves very much. How do you think this ultimately affects a friendship?
5. Is it a sign of a good friendship that the friends never have any conflict with each other?
6. Have you ever had a conflict with a friend that resulted in the friendship being stronger than it was before? What made it stronger?

II. Conflicts in Friendships (25 min.)

For this small group activity, each group will work on an idea that the larger group comes up with as a "common problem" in friendships. Generate ideas by saying to the students:

> *We are going to get into small groups and try to come up with ideas for ways to solve some problems that are common in friendships. Let's try to think of 5 to 6 conflict scenarios that frequently happen in*

friendships and write them on the board. Each group will spend some time brainstorming ideas for ways to solve the problem.

After the students have thought of 5 to 6 ideas, break the students into small groups with a leader, reporter, recorder, and group members. Each group will be given one of the scenarios in which conflict has occurred in a friendship. Ask the students to brainstorm as many solutions to this conflict as they can think of, and ask them to write them down on their handout.

After about 7–10 minutes, reconvene the groups, and ask each group to share its scenarios and solutions to the problems. Discuss how some solutions may work better than others, how some solutions make things worse. Discuss how RAID and SCIDDLE have been used in some situations to resolve conflict.

III. Tenkan—The Art of Listening (15 min.)

One theme that is most likely to run through many of the solutions the students came up with will be the *importance of listening to our friends when we are in a conflict with them.* Summarize how this came out in the small groups in your own words:

> *One theme that I heard in many of the ideas you shared was the importance of listening to our friends when we are in a conflict with them. For example, in this small group over here. . . .*

Explain that one way to be a good friend is to do the things you want your friends to do to you:

As you probably know, one of the best ways to have good friends is to be a good friend. In other words, if we want someone to treat us a certain way, we should treat them the way we want to be treated. Do you agree? Why or why not?

After discussing this principle of reciprocity, apply it to listening by introducing the Tenkan activity:

> *In the case of being a good listener, one way we can treat the other person as we want to be treated is this:* **when we have conflict in our friendships we can be the first one to start listening.** *I have an activity I want us to try called Tenkan. Can I have a volunteer please?*

Explain to the volunteer that you will be grabbing onto his or her wrist and that you want the person to argue with you about what is in the room. You will argue by saying that the room has the things in it you see behind the student's head; the student will argue by saying the room has the things in it he or she sees behind your head. You will pull each other back and forth for a while and then ask the audience if you are getting anywhere. For example,

"I told you, the room has a door and a pencil sharpener and a teacher's desk!"

"I don't think so! There's no teacher's desk! The room is full of student desks and a TV/VCR!"

"Right, you idiot! You're seeing things!"

and so on. . . .

After asking the class how this is working, repeat the dispute, but after a couple of interchanges, take a step in toward the student volunteer, stand next to him or her, face the same way, and put your arm around his or her shoulders. Say loudly and with enthusiasm, something like, "Oh my goodness, you are right! There ARE a bunch of student desks and a TV/VCR. I didn't see that before." Then, take a step to spin the student volunteer around to see your side of the room. Say something like, "Oh, and I want to show you something. Look, see how from my perspective there's just a desk and a pencil sharpener. Isn't that amazing?! We both were right!"

After doing this demonstration, ask the students what the "lesson" is:

OK, so you saw this activity called Tenkan. What is the lesson from this activity?

Once the students seem to understand how both sides of an argument can be right and that listening to our friends can help us look at things differently, ask them to stand up and try the *Tenkan* activity a few times themselves with a partner. Remind them to be safe! Encourage them to role-play the dispute as well as the "listening."

After about four minutes, when everyone has had a chance to try both roles, ask the students to return to their seats.

IV. Closure (10 min.)

Ask them the following question about friendship and write their ideas on the board:

Now we have had some practice with one important quality in friendships—that of being a good listener. Let's make a list of other characteristics we would look for in our friendships, and I will write them on the board.

After the students have created a long list, remind them of the saying, "To make a good friend is to be a good friend. Ask them to go around the group and complete the sentence,

"One thing I look for in my friendships that I do myself is. . . . "

WORKING IN SMALL GROUPS

Friendship and Conflict

Leader

Go over the assignment with the group:
1. Remind the group of the conflict assigned to their group.
2. Make a list of the things people could do if they had this conflict with a friend.
3. Make sure everyone participates.
4. Be sure the group is done in six minutes.

Group Members

Think of as many ways as possible to solve the conflict in the friendship.

Recorder

Write down the conflict and the solutions below.

Reporter

Read the group's conflict and solutions to the large group.

1. One common conflict that occurs in friendships is. . . .

2. Possible solutions to this conflict are. . . .

Instructional Resource Page for Session 4

Physical Contact. In this session, the activity "Tenkan" provides a concrete example of the validity of opposing points of view because it provides visual proof of the truth of both viewpoints. Ideally, every student will be able to participate in this activity once the volunteers have demonstrated. However, because there is physical contact between students, special care should be taken to make sure the activity is carried out appropriately. For example, it may be helpful to have a limited number of student pairs experimenting with the activity at a time.

7

Overview of RIPP-8

This chapter provides an overview of RIPP-8, the 12-session violence prevention curriculum designed for the third year of either middle school (8th grade) or junior high school (9th grade). Once the essence and core components of RIPP-8 are described, a description of the strategies used in the program is presented. A short summary of the goals for each session is provided, as well as a sample session. The standardized RIPP-8 instructor manual (approximately 100 pages) is available through the Life Skills Center and is intended to be used in tandem with the guidance in operations and evaluation that is provided in this monograph.

THE ESSENCE OF RIPP-8

The essence of the final year of RIPP is to make the transition to high school an opportunity for promoting nonviolence by facilitating positive risk-taking in youth. Although adolescent risk-taking is often perceived as having negative consequences, we believe this desire for challenge can be tapped for the benefit of youth and their communities. By challenge we refer to activities such as imagining the future, setting personal goals, making new friends, forgiving someone who has hurt you, working hard in school, applying for a job, choosing nonviolence, and making a positive difference in the community.

Instead of introducing a new acronym for RIPP-8, we decided that it would be helpful for students to use their improved cognitive abilities to take a closer look at the skills they have learned in RIPP. For example, when coping with challenges is addressed, students learn that SCIDDLE contains strategies for both problem-focused coping (e.g., Decide among your options, Evaluate) and emotion-focused coping (e.g., Calm down, Identify your feelings).

EDUCATIONAL STRATEGIES AND CONTENT

The key addition used in RIPP-8 in terms of educational strategies is an activity designed by Dr. Tom Smith, a leader in outdoor adventure, who recently received the Kurt Hahn Leadership Award for lifetime contributions to the field. His activity, the Raccoon Circle, builds on the symbolic meaning of the circle (e.g., unity, connectedness, community) and uses the circle in group activities (Smith, 1996). The Raccoon Circle is a webbing 10–12 feet long that is knotted into a circle of a 4–5 feet in diameter. The circle is used in a variety of activities and games that rely on group cohesion and unity. Ideally, the Raccoon Circle and information-sharing activities promote positive risk-taking in a safe and supportive environment.

12 SESSIONS OF RIPP-8

RIPP-8 consists of 12 fifty-minute sessions that are to be taught weekly, beginning in the second half of the school year. Following is a short description of the goals for each session.

Session 1: Introduction and Review

The goals of this session are to reintroduce the purpose of the RIPP program and to develop group cohesion by establishing ground rules.

Session 2: Stereotypes

The goal of this lesson is to point out to students the destructive nature of stereotypes for others and for themselves. Stereotyping happens when we do not listen to the facts about ourselves and others.

Session 3: Attitude

The goals of this session are to review and practice working in small groups, to help students understand how attitudes can influence both perceptions about people (stereotypes) and perceptions about situations, and to show how our attitude can influence our stress level and our health.

Session 4: Choosing the Big Picture

The goal of this session is to demonstrate how being open-minded and looking at various solutions and viewpoints helps a person deal with others in a non-violent way. RAID options are an example of the bigger picture.

Session 5: Emotion-Focused Coping

This session provides an opportunity for students to think about ways to respond when they are faced with a problem that they either have no power to change or are too upset about to deal with constructively. Positive strategies of emotion-focused coping are discussed and practiced.

Session 6: Problem-Focused Coping

In this session, students see how SCIDDLE is made up of both emotion-focused coping and problem-focused coping.

Session 7: Risk-Taking

The goal of this session is to help students differentiate between positive and negative risk-taking and the subsequent outcomes.

Session 8: Envisioning the Future—Positive Risk-Taking

The goals of this session are to expand on the idea of positive risk-taking and to help students apply this when thinking of future and immediate goals (i.e., high school goals).

Session 9: Expanding on RAID with Forgiveness

Because many students are either victims of violence or exposed to it, this session focuses on constructive ways to respond. The option of forgiveness is introduced, and students are challenged to consider this as a positive risk they may want to take.

Session 10: Envisioning the Future—Create Your Job

The goals of this session are to introduce the idea that we can use our personal strengths and future education to prepare us for work that will be satisfying and pay well. Students begin to generate ideas for ways they can make high school an opportunity to gain the experience and skills they need.

Session 11: Envisioning the Future— What About Everyone Else?

The goals of this session are to help students understand what is most important to them and how their actions influence others. A specific focus is made on the relationship between having positive goals and community violence.

Session 12: Your Future

The goal of this final session is for students to create a "Tree of Life" that represents their future ideal, their values, and the actions they will take in high school to help them actualize their future.

SAMPLE SESSION

Session 9: Expanding on RAID with Forgiveness

Goal

Because many students are either victims of violence or are exposed to it, this session focuses on constructive ways to respond. The option of forgiveness is introduced, and students are challenged to consider this as a positive risk they may want to take.

Key Concepts

- Forgiveness: Letting go of negative feelings toward a person who wronged you and replacing them with positive feelings, a sense of well-wishing, and maybe a desire to reconcile, if safe and possible.
- Revenge: Making something bad happen, or wishing it would, to a person who wronged you.
- Forgetting: A way to protect yourself from negative feelings toward the person who wronged you by refusing to admit a feeling; includes denial and/or acceptance.

Materials and Preparation:

- Prepare a personal scenario for use in practicing forgiveness.
- Remember one time you chose forgiveness that you can share with students.

CLASSROOM ACTIVITIES

I. Review (3 minutes)

Provide an introduction to today's topic by reviewing the last workshop:

We've been talking about things we can change and things we cannot change because we don't have control over them. Today we will spend more time on things we don't have control over. We are going to focus especially on options we have if we are victims of violence or have seen it (been exposed to it). What are some examples?

II. Forgiveness, Revenge, and Forgetting (9 minutes)

Write each of the following three words on the board and ask the students to define them: forgiveness, revenge, and forgetting. After the students have defined the words, share the definitions provided in the key concepts for this session.

After defining the words, create three columns on the board, one each for the three terms. Ask the students to respond to the following questions for each:

1. When might I want to do this?
2. How does it feel to do this? In the short term? In the long term?
3. What are the benefits of this? The costs?
4. What is the relationship of this to violence? The web of violence? The web of support?

III. Practicing Forgiveness (12 minutes)

In this activity, you will share a model for forgiveness and apply it to a situation you are currently working on. This scenario should be something you are genuinely dealing with, yet something you feel comfortable sharing with the group.

Explain the model for forgiveness:

Just as we have a problem-solving model for conflict called SCIDDLE, there is a problem-solving model for forgiveness called REACH. This model was developed by Dr. Everett Worthington, an internationally recognized leader in research on forgiveness. REACH stands for:

- *Recall and acknowledge the hurt*
- *Empathize (imagine the other person's perspective)*
- *Altruistic gift (recall when you have been forgiven by another, what was that feeling like—can you give it to another person?)*
- *Commit to your choice (formal action that includes letting go, positive feelings, and clarifying boundaries of the relationship in a way that is good for you)*
- *Hold on to your choice (all components—letting go, positive feelings, and clarified boundaries)*

Now, let's apply these steps to a problem that I am dealing with right now. . .

Share your situation and then ask the students to help you apply each of the steps to your situation. Once you are complete, thank the students for assisting you with this.

IV. Connecting Forgiveness to SCIDDLE and RAID (5 minutes)

Ask the students the following questions to help them draw connections between forgiveness, SCIDDLE, and RAID:

- Which parts of SCIDDLE does forgiveness connect to? Which parts of RAID?
- How does forgiveness relate to the E-step of SCIDDLE?
- Is forgiveness a choice? When might you choose this? Why?

V. Closure: Challenge to Try the Positive Risk of Forgiveness (10 minutes)

Begin this activity by sharing a time when you chose forgiveness that resulted in positive consequences for you:

One time I tried forgiveness that worked well for me is . . .

After you have shared your experience, challenge the students to consider using this positive risk. Ask them to pair off and share one thing they learned today about forgiveness:

I realize that forgiveness isn't something new for you, but I would like to challenge you to try using this positive risk. Now, I'd like you to pair off and share one thing you've learned today about forgiveness.

Instructional Resource for Session 9

Forgiveness as a Social-Cognitive Skill. Because the word *forgiveness* may bring to mind worries about bringing religion into the classroom, it is important to recognize that it represents a synthesis of many of the social-cognitive skills taught in RIPP. For example, forgiveness involves calming down, imagining the other person's perspective, listening to what is important to you, defining what is safe for you, valuing the friendship, and staying focused on the problem, not the person.

8

Adaptation of RIPP For Cultural and Community Differences

OVERVIEW

In the previous chapters we've discussed the implementation and evaluation of RIPP in an urban and a rural school system. Will RIPP work in other communities? This is a particularly important question for those who are considering implementing RIPP in their community. Although RIPP was developed for a primarily low-income, urban, African-American population, RIPP is not a culture-specific program. This is evidenced by our ability to successfully adapt this program to a vastly different student population in a rural system. Similarly, although RIPP has been evaluated with high-risk populations, the program is not restricted to such populations. The recent outbreak of school shootings in communities considered low-risk, such as Littleton, Colorado, and Jonesboro, Arkansas, has raised our nation's awareness of the need for violence prevention programs across communities of varying risk levels. Increasingly, schools across the country are realizing the need to address the issue of violence, as well as develop school norms for nonviolence. We believe that the theoretical model upon which RIPP is based and the intervention techniques will be an appropriate violence prevention program for middle and junior high schools that represent different types of communities, cultures, and risk levels.

At the same time, it would be naïve to believe that one could simply pick up the RIPP manual and apply the program without considering the characteristics of the intended community. Even if the program were implemented in another urban community, schools within that community would probably differ in sig-

97

nificant ways from the urban community in which RIPP was developed. Such differences might relate to school size, the presence or absence of gangs within the schools, the degree of heterogeneity in the student population, structural issues (e.g., school locations), the distance students travel to schools, the presence of other programs, and school disciplinary policies. The RIPP program follows the recommendations of others in the prevention area who believe that a program should begin with a strong theoretical model and empirically tested methods and then adapt specific components to the intended population (Coatsworth, Szapocznik, Kurtines, & Santisban, 1997; Yung & Hammond, 1998).

Adapting programs is a significant issue that should be thought out critically and done in consultation with a knowledgeable group such as the management team (discussed in Chapter 2). In particular, close attention should be paid to cultural and community influences in developing and maintaining violence in the target community. This chapter discusses ideas to consider when adapting RIPP to specific communities. We begin with a discussion of ways the theoretical basis of RIPP can guide adaptations to the program. Then, we outline some of the major research findings on characteristics of different communities and populations that might play a role in developing and maintaining of violence. Specifically, we discuss issues of community context, school environment, ethnicity, and gender. Next, we describe how to use the theoretical basis of RIPP to adapt specific components of the program and provide examples of adaptations we have made to the RIPP program in urban and rural schools.

THEORETICAL BASIS OF RIPP

As previously described, RIPP is based on social-cognitive learning theory (Bandura, 1986, 1989) which purports that violence is the result of a complex set of interactive relationships that exist between the person, the behavior, and the environment. In this view, the individual and the environment share the responsibility when aggression occurs. Unfortunately, when violence occurs, we often try to find someone to blame. Some blame the perpetrator, whereas others look to the parents or peer group. Still others believe that the school, legal system, or community is at fault. Social-cognitive learning theory purports that all of these factors play a role to some degree because children develop and actively interact in a complex social system that includes parents, peers, the school, and the community.

Consistent with this view, RIPP is designed to address individual, behavioral, and environmental factors that are particularly relevant to youth in middle/ junior high schools. In addition, RIPP targets the types of violence that are most likely to be evident during adolescence—situational and interpersonal violence. Situational violence stems primarily from environmental factors such as school norms, poverty, neighborhood norms, and availability of handguns; interpersonal violence results from disputes between individuals who have an ongoing relationship (Tolan & Guerra, 1994). A quick examination of the 12 objectives of the RIPP program (see Chapter 1) shows how we articulated the ways in which RIPP can affect these types of violence by addressing the three domains of environment, individual factors, and behaviors. For example, Objective 1 (Develop norms and expectations for nonviolent means of conflict resolution and positive achievement) helps to reduce environmental factors that can escalate an interpersonal dispute into situational violence. Whereas this objective may be the same at all schools that implement RIPP, the exact language that expresses these norms and how they relate to cultural norms about nonviolence may vary from community to community, as well as within communities. Therefore, an understanding of the community, school, and students can guide adaptations for "Making RIPP Real" for a specific school. The following section describes a number of dimensions in which communities differ from each other that can help promote consideration of what is special about a particular community.

COMMUNITY AND CULTURAL INFLUENCES ON VIOLENCE

Multiple factors contribute to violence, and one characteristic is rarely enough to predict whether violence will occur. For example, it is often noted that rates of crime and violence are generally higher among African-Americans than among other ethnic groups in the United States (Hamburg, 1998). However, evidence suggests that poverty and living in a low-income neighborhood are more strongly related to violence than ethnicity (Lowry, Sleet, Duncan, Powell, & Kolbe, 1995). The reason for the disproportionately high rates of violence among African-Americans may be because African-Americans are more likely to be in poverty, often because perceived racism or lack of opportunities fuel the cycle of poverty (Sampson, 1993). "Perceived racism" refers to both objective experiences of racism, as well as other more subjective actions that may be viewed by an individual as racism. Such subjective experiences are no less stressful to the individual than the objective experiences (Clark, Anderson, Clark, & Williams, 1999). At the same time, poverty alone is not predictive of violence but becomes significant only when it occurs along with other community attributes (Laub & Lauritsen, 1998). Another example of multiple factors that contribute to violence is that certain behaviors may have vastly different meanings, depending on the cultural group or community. For example, carrying a gun in an urban area is generally associated with violent activity. On the other hand, guns in rural areas are typically used for hunting. Such complex interactions must be considered when evaluating violence within specific communities and among specific cultures.

To begin making sense of such interactions in a particular community, the management team should first evaluate aspects of the school, community, and students to understand potential risk and protective factors for violence. The management team should also consider potential issues of concern in implementing a violence prevention program. The team may wish to consult with teachers, parents, and students through surveys and/or focus groups. It is important to elicit different viewpoints to gain a more complete picture. Students, for example, may have vastly different views on the issues relating to violence than their parents, teachers, or school administrators. It is also important to gain input from a range of sources. For example, opinions should be obtained from a representative sample of students, not just those who are considered leaders. Some potential issues to consider include, but are not limited to, the following:

- What is the type of community (urban, rural, or suburban)? How is this community similar to and different from others of the same type (e.g., if it is an urban community, how does it compare to other urban communities?).
- Is the surrounding neighborhood generally safe, or are there problems with crime and violence? Do most of the students come from the surrounding neighborhoods, or are they bused in from different communities? Are the students exposed to crime and violence outside of school?
- What is the socioeconomic status (SES) of the students? Are most students from the same SES or is there variability?
- Are gangs a problem in the community? Are they a problem in the school?
- Do students and teachers feel safe at school? Do students get involved in physical altercations at school? Have teachers been threatened by students?
- How is status achieved at school? What are the different types of peer groups, and how do they relate to each other? Are some students socially rejected or bullied?
- What is the ethnic composition of the school? How do the students relate to or feel about students from different ethnic groups?
- How do boys and girls display aggression? For example, are disciplinary problems and violent encounters more common among boys than girls, or do both genders display such problem behaviors?

Along with answering such questions, the management team should consider how such characteristics influence the presence or absence of violence in the school and community. The following sections will attempt to clarify some of the multiple community and cultural influences on violence that interact together with the individual to encourage or discourage violent occurrences. Our discussion of these issues is not meant to be exhaustive or prescriptive but rather to provide readers with issues to consider in implementing RIPP in their own communities.

Community Context

There are vast differences in rates of crime and violence by community context. One of the most influential theories of why such differences occur is social disorganization theory (Shaw & McKay, 1969). This theory argues that communities that are more disorganized will tend to have higher rates of crime and violence. In such communities, residents have fewer resources and social ties, which in turn prohibits residents from exerting informal social controls over delinquency and violence. Community characteristics associated with social disorganization include poverty and economic deprivation, a high percentage of single adult heads of households, high divorce rates, high population density, high population turnover, and ethnic heterogeneity. These individual factors by themselves do not lead to violence but are related to social disorganization. Such a theory moves us away from simple explanations of violence. For example, it is not sufficient to say that poverty leads to violence because there are neighborhoods that are relatively poor, but are stable, and are therefore able to exert informal social control. Likewise, ethnic minorities are not necessarily more violent, but ethnic heterogeneity is highly correlated with rates of growth and change, which are associated with social disorganization (Laub & Lauritsen, 1998).

Urban Neighborhoods

Researchers examining neighborhood factors in violence have noted that urban neighborhoods often have significantly higher rates of crime and other social problems than other areas. Children in inner city neighborhoods often witness or are victims of violence. As many as 70% of inner city youths have been victimized by violent acts, and 85% of these youth report witnessing violence in their neighborhoods (Fitzpatrick & Boldizar, 1993). Such neighborhoods tend to be plagued by a high amount of social disorganization, including low socioeconomic status and a high residential turnover (Shaw & McKay, 1969).

Violence in these communities may be seen as a goal-oriented behavior in that violence may be used to achieve and maintain social status, obtain material goods, and obtain social justice. Violence may also be used for self-protection and as a way to defy authority. In the absence of opportunities for good jobs and the lack of role models within the community who have achieved status through work, violence becomes a way to achieve status in the community that is often supported by neighborhood norms (Wilson, 1987). Likewise, the poverty of inner cities creates an environment in which there is a stark contrast between having and not having, but where it may be extremely difficult for many individuals to procure material things legally (Fagan & Wilkinson, 1998).

Gangs may exist in both large and small cities and consist of various ethnic compositions. Like violence itself, the presence of gangs in a community is linked more to a lack of social control than the type of community or ethnicity. In socially and economically isolated communities, gangs may provide their members with a sense of belonging and opportunities for financial gain through robberies and drug sales (Fagan, 1999). Violence is an intrinsic part of gangs and often considered part of the gang's collective identity (Padilla, 1992). Gang violence can be seen as purposeful and organized. Violence may occur in power struggles within the gang, territorial battles with other gangs, gang rituals, status attainment, material gain, and retribution and self-defense of the members or the gang as a whole (Fagan & Wilkinson, 1998).

Rural Neighborhoods

Although much of the focus of social disorganization has been on urban areas, rural neighborhoods are often characterized by disorganization as well. Poverty is often a significant problem in rural areas that contributes significantly to health problems (Human & Wassem, 1991). Research has documented increasing trends in antisocial behavior among rural youth and has implicated economic stress among rural families as a key contributor (Conger & Elder, 1994). In the rural school system where we implemented RIPP, there is a large percentage of migrant workers. The percentage of migrant workers contributes to high residential turnover, associated with social disorganization. Along with economic hardships, this instability of the population is likely to contribute to social disorganization. In turn, such social disorganization may have been the reason that we found such high rates of students reporting being both witnesses and perpetrators of violence among rural students.

Suburban Neighborhoods

Suburban areas are often considered stable and secure places. People often "escape" to the suburbs to avoid the crime associated with urban areas. However, as the recent shooting in Littleton, Colorado, illustrated, suburban schools are not immune to violent occurrences. The outbreak of school violence in stable suburban areas has been especially puzzling because crime rates in these neighborhoods are generally low. Suburban neighborhoods are not associated with poverty or high residential turnover rates that have been linked to social disorganization. However, suburban neighborhoods may have disorganizational characteristics that may prevent community interaction. Suburban neighborhoods are often comprised of residents who have much in common (such as socioeconomic level and ethnicity) and yet may have little interaction or involvement with one another because the neighborhoods are relatively new (and thus don't have a community "history"). This isolation can be compounded if large numbers of adolescents are left at home unsupervised by parents who commute great distances to work. In addition, in wealthier suburban communities, neighbors may unintentionally set up social norms that promote a sense of competition between neighbors. These social norms may also promote an "us versus them" mentality that hinders the development of acceptance of differences among neighbors (e.g., differences in socioeconomic status and ethnicity) (Warren & Warren, 1977). Adolescents may model and promote the community social norm of competitiveness and stereotyping with neighborhood and school peers, which in turn may promote hostility and aggression. Furthermore, it is important to note that although schools often reflect the larger neighborhood and community, this is not always the case. The school itself might set up informal social norms that unintentionally promote violence.

School Environment

It is generally believed that school violence reflects violence in the broader social context. Indeed, this is often the case. Schools in violent neighborhoods generally have more problems with violence than those in safer neighborhoods because violence is imported to the school through the students and others who reside in the neighborhood (Reiss & Roth, 1993). However, the school itself might create a unique environment. Such an environment might work for or against the best interests of the students. For example, a school climate that values individuals and promotes attitudes and behaviors that respect and protect the rights of others provides a significant protective factor through bonding to the school (Remboldt, 1998). Such bonding occurs by having ample opportunities to be active in the educational process, developing skills necessary for success in school, and receiving reinforcement for school involvement and successes. At the same time, school bonding alone is not enough to prevent violence. Along with creating the appropriate circumstances for bonding to occur, schools need to actively promote nonviolence (Hawkins, Farrington, & Catalano, 1998).

In contrast, a school climate that operates by intimidation and provides few role models of prosocial behavior and little institutional support for positive conflict resolution may foster violence (Meyer & Northup, 1997). Schools may unintentionally create a social context for violence. Students, often from diverse backgrounds, spend considerable time at school in close proximity to their classmates. Students often compete for status within the school. Violence may be used in such circumstances to gain social status and correct perceived injustices (Elliot, Hamburg, & Williams, 1998; Remboldt, 1998). This may be compounded when neighborhood norms also support the use of aggression for status or justice. In economically stressed communities, prosocial means of achieving status (e.g., school success, employment) might be limited because of the lack of opportunities or negative attitudes toward such goals (Fagan & Wilkinson, 1998). Additionally, schools that do not adequately protect their students from victimization may unintentionally promote violence. Children who are repeatedly victimized often become the perpetrators of violence (Olweaus, 1978). Children who feel unsafe at school may carry weapons such as knives or guns as a way to protect themselves, leading to reactive aggression (Loeber & Stouthamer-Loeber, 1998).

Schools may also provide opportunities to learn violent behaviors through associations with deviant peers because schools are often the place where friendships are developed. The confluence hypothesis (Dishion, Patterson, & Griesler, 1994) helps to explain how both individual and environmental factors contribute to the development of deviant friendships and the "training" of deviant behaviors through these friendships. This hypothesis suggests that children who display antisocial behavior (e.g., delinquency, aggression) are likely to be rejected by the majority of their peers. They select friends who also display antisocial behavior because of this limited pool of potential friends, as well as the tendency to select friends based on similar values and interests. School policies may further contribute to deviant children selecting deviant friends. Classes are often created based on ability level and/or behavioral problems which increases the chances that these children will develop friendships with peers similar in these respects (Kellam, 1990). Once such friendships are formed they tend to reinforce antisocial behaviors, and new antisocial values and behaviors may be formed in the context of such friendships, a process Dishion et al. (1994) call "deviancy training."

Ethnicity

Ethnic minority groups in the United States are disproportionately represented as both victims and perpetrators of violence. This is particularly true for African-Americans. For example, homicide is the second leading cause of death among 15 to 24-year-olds in the United States. However, when you look specifically at African-Americans, homicide is the leading cause of death among this age group (Hawkins, Crosby, & Hammett, 1994). Does it then follow that *being* African-American in and of itself increases the risk of violent behavior? In other words, is there something inherent in ethnicity that contributes to violent behavior? The answer is likely no because the high rates of violence among African-Americans in the United States seem to be specific to the American culture. For example, Black females and males who live in other countries that are homogeneous (e.g., Nigeria) or predominantly White (e.g., Canada) do not have unusually high rates of violent offending (Kruttschnitt, 1995). Risk factors for violence in this country have included unemployment, high population density, and poverty. The higher level of these risk factors among ethnic minorities than among Whites is a viable explanation for the higher rates of violence among minorities. Furthermore, the perceived racism, discrimination, and inequality that may be experienced by ethnic minorities contribute significantly to a cycle of poverty and violence (Sampson, 1993).

A discussion of ethnic minorities would not be complete without some acknowledgement of the long history of discrimination they have endured in this country (see Axelson, 1993 and Hill, Soriano, Chen, & LaFrambrose, 1994 for a more complete review). For example, at one point in this country's history, Native Americans and their culture were systematically destroyed. Native Americans were forced to move to substandard housing on reservations, prevented from engaging in cultural rituals, and had their children taken away from them to be "reeducated" in boarding schools. Many African-Americans were brought to this country involuntarily as slaves and did not begin to gain full rights as citizens until the Civil Rights movement in the 1960s (Axelson, 1993). Racism and discrimination against these and other ethnic minority groups have led to a lack of educational and employment opportunities that have prevented social and economic growth among many. Even minority groups that are considered economically successful have experienced considerable discrimination. Asians have been called the "model minority," yet the immigration laws that exist today were originally created to keep Chinese from entering the country. Moreover, during World War II, Japanese-Americans, even those born in this country, were sent to concentration camps as war criminals. Furthermore, both Asian immigrants from other countries and Asian-Americans are often accused of stealing jobs and monopolizing business opportunities (Hill et al., 1994), which can escalate conflict among ethnic groups.

Although ethnic minorities have many more legal rights today than they had in the past, discrimination and racism may persist in more insidious ways. For example, the very poverty experienced by minorities that has been linked to the longstanding history of discrimination has been used to justify viewing minorities as "lazy." Moreover, the apparently positive stereotype of Asians being economically successful may result in discrimination and lack of services to those Asians who do experience economic adversity and unemployment (Hill et al., 1994). It is the interactive relationship between such stereotypes and discrimination, limited access to resources, and lack of economic resources necessary to meet the basic standards of living of a particular society or location that seem to account for the levels of violence among ethnic minorities (Sampson, 1993).

Thus far we have been speaking in generalities about ethnic minorities. It is important to note that there are considerable differences within groups of ethnic minorities. Many individuals with ethnic minority backgrounds, often with poor backgrounds, have gained economic and social success in this country even in the face of adversity. In fact, there are values embedded in many ethnic cultures that may serve to protect individuals from violent risk factors. Generally speaking, Latino culture emphasizes the importance of family, respect for authority figures, and a reverence for peace. Similarly, African-American culture stresses the importance of harmony and respect for life, as well as spirituality (see McGoldrick, Pearce, & Giordano, 1982 for a more complete discussion of values among ethnic cultures and among subgroups of such cultures).

Such values may protect individuals from risk factors in engaging in violent acts but as a whole have generally been unsuccessful in protecting the entire culture. In some cases, cultural values have been so belittled or actively destroyed (as with Native Americans) that the youth no longer identify with them. Another potential problem arises when cultural values are upheld within a context where norms exist that support violence. For example, the Latino values around family may draw youth to gangs as surrogate families. Additionally, reverence for authority could be applied to delinquent or violent leaders (Hill et al., 1994). Oliver (1989) lists several other reasons that cultural values have failed to impact the level of violence among ethnic minorities. Specifically, the risk factors may outweigh the potential protective qualities; youth may get mixed messages from their own culture and the mainstream culture and not be able to disentangle them; youth may not be equipped to deal with the conflict between cultural and mainstream values and thus may adopt street or other delinquent values; and finally, cultures may adopt maladaptive strategies to achieve power and efficacy because they cannot be achieved through prosocial means.

Gender

It has been suggested that boys and girls differ in the way they express aggression. Previous research has tended to focus on the physical aggression that is most common among boys. Nonphysical aggression includes relational aggression that aims to damage a person through peer relationships (e.g., excluding someone from a group, spreading a rumor), and has been identified as particularly salient for girls (Crick & Grotpeter, 1995). Research (Crick, Bigbee, & Howes, 1996; Crick & Grotpeter, 1995) has consistently shown that girls tend to engage in relational aggression more so than boys; that relational aggression is more common in girls' same-sex peer groups; and that friendships among highly relationally aggressive girls involve higher levels of intimacy, jealousy, and exclusivity. Research has also suggested that nonnormative aggressive behaviors (e.g., physical aggression in girls) may result in more severe maladjustment outcomes than either normative aggression or nonaggression (Crick, 1997). It is important to note, however, that other types of nonphysical aggression such as verbal aggression (e.g., insults) may be used equally by both boys and girls (Lagerspetz, Bjorkqvist, & Paltonen, 1988). In addition, gender differences in relational and physical aggression may vary by culture (Tomada & Schneider, 1997).

The different ways of expressing aggression among boys and girls might explain why previous research that has tended to focus on physical forms of aggression has found higher prevalence rates for boys than girls. However, other factors such as community context and ethnicity might play a role as well. In our examinations of the urban self-report data, we typically find few differences between boys and girls in physical aggression. In a recent study, we found that boys and girls tended to be more similar in the urban schools than in the rural schools in physical aggression items (Farrell, Kung, White, & Valois, in press). Because samples differed in several respects (e.g., setting, ethnicity, region, grade level), it is not clear which factor or factors were responsible for these observed differences. These findings suggest, however, that gender differences might vary according to one or more factors.

Children with Learning and/or Behavioral Disorders

Students with special educational needs, such as those with learning disorders or behavioral or emotional disorders, pose a challenge in most classroom settings. RIPP facilitators may find themselves in classrooms with one or two "mainstreamed" special education students, or they may be assigned to a special education class.To help facilitators effectively apply the RIPP program in these situations, a description of the specific challenges of working with special education children should be presented during training, as well as potential strategies for applying the RIPP program.

Students who have learning difficulties are typically believed to have a structural or ability deficit that prevents them from understanding core concepts presented in the classroom. However, although these deficits may exist, research suggests that difficulties in self-regulation and organization may be the key factor in these children's poor performance. Aside from poor academic performance, other characteristics associated with children who have learning disabilities include helpless behavior, low motivation, low productivity, and impulsivity. In addition, children who have learning disabilities often have difficulty understanding the association between saying and doing and therefore find it difficult to use verbalizations to guide their behavior (Wong, Harris, & Graham, 1991).

Because behavior, affect, and cognitions are integrally related, learning and behavior difficulties often go hand in hand. Children with emotional or behavioral disorders often display uncooperative behaviors in the classroom and have difficulty working with their peers. They often fail to develop positive interpersonal relationships with teachers, administrators, and other students. However, research indicates that the development of such relationships is crucial to their academic achievement and future development (Cartledge & Cochran, 1993). Cooperative learning, in which children work together in small groups to achieve a certain goal, may promote positive peer interactions, increase academic achievement, and improve self-esteem. Therefore, the RIPP format of small group work has a potential to be especially beneficial to special education children.

ADAPTING RIPP

The community and cultural issues that should be considered in adapting RIPP underscore the necessity of having the management team review the characteristics of their own school and community and consider ways in which these characteristics might influence program content and implementation. As mentioned previously, it is vital that any adaptations be critically thought out and not done simply for convenience. Adapting programs is a tricky issue, and it is often difficult to find the right balance between being overly focused on the unique characteristics of a group and deviating too much from the manual and being too worried about following the program manual and not making necessary changes. Some general advice is to consider the general framework the manual provides as well as the match between a particular population and the content of the manual (Addis, Hatgis, Soysa, Zaslavsky, & Bourne, 1999). More specifically, consider the framework and objectives of the RIPP program and how the workshops outlined in the manual fit into this framework and meet specific objectives. Then consider how these workshops might be adapted to meet the needs of a specific population, still fit into the overall framework, and meet the program objectives.

In this section, we outline particular issues in adapting RIPP to new communities. This begins with a discussion of issues in adapting program components. Throughout our discussion, we include relevant examples of adjustments we have made in our urban and rural populations. Because it is important to follow the original program as closely as possible to achieve similar results, the particular adaptations provided here follow the general framework of RIPP and meet the program objectives. They are provided to give clear examples of modifying an activity for a specific audience while maintaining the integrity of the goals for the activity.

Program Components

As mentioned previously, RIPP is not a culturally specific program. The skills taught in each session are relevant to a wide array of students. At the same time, the details included in the sessions, the language used, and who teaches the program are likely to vary by community. Whenever a person contemplates a change in the program, he or she should review the purpose of the original activities and make sure that the modifications are true to the original intent.

Sessions

It is important to make RIPP "real" to the students by drawing from current, applicable, and culturally relevant situations and occurrences. On a general level, it is important for the facilitator to keep abreast of local incidents so that he or she can integrate them into RIPP when appropriate. In terms of specific change, consider the first workshop of the 6th grade program as an example. The "Find Someone Who" activity could easily be adjusted to different communities. In the urban schools, where the majority of students are African-American, we include culturally specific items such as "likes African dance," and "celebrates Kwaanza with their family." These items were not as appropriate for students living in a rural area, where the population is much more heterogeneous, and were therefore replaced with other items such as "likes fishing in Lake Okeechobee." In the second workshop, the FBI should be contacted to find local statistics for the homicide worksheet (304-625-2000). In workshop 16, the facilitator should review how the "civil rights" story played out for the various ethnic groups represented in the class. An example would be how Cesar Chavez fought for migrant farm workers' rights. During the Values Voting activity in workshop 20, students could be encouraged to choose statements that reflect biases in their own ethnic group. In addition, the 7th and 8th grade booster sessions use various scenarios between friends and family for classroom exercises; these scenarios can be easily changed to fit the climate of the school and community. Such adjustments do not take away from the overall message of RIPP but make the program more accessible and meaningful to the target population.

Adding or substituting session components may also help facilitate the students' understanding of the material, so long as such components are consistent with the overall framework or specific objectives of RIPP. In the rural schools, for example, one of the facilitators came across a video that addressed the negative consequences of violence. This video seemed appropriate to add to the RIPP program because it fit with the goal of Session 2 to increase students' awareness of the impact that violence can have on the quality of life. On the other hand, a facilitator in an urban school wanted to include a discussion of the reality of death. His reason was that the students in the community were exposed to such high rates of violence and that several had experienced the death of someone they knew through violent means. However, we felt that discussing death as part of the RIPP program would be likely to lead to normalizing the experiences of death, which is not consistent with any of the program objectives.

Language

To successfully complete the RIPP program, the participants will need to be relatively proficient in the language used. It obviously doesn't make sense to administer the program in English to Spanish-speaking students. Beyond general understanding, the students also need to relate to the language used. The RIPP program avoids technical terms and attempts to use language that youth will understand. However, different communities and cultures have expressions and slang words that might be unique to them. The inclusion of such community or culturally specific expressions might help the students better relate to the role-plays and messages of RIPP. However, it is not appropriate to use profanity or to use expressions that either glorify or normalize violence, no matter how prevalent in the community.

Facilitator

The facilitator is an important role model and it is imperative that the facilitator be a person with whom the students can relate. Some programs recommend that the facilitator be matched to the characteristics of the participants. In other words, if the participants are primarily African-American, an African-American facilitator should implement the program (Yung & Hammond, 1998). We have not specified the ethnicity of the facilitator but rather have looked for candidates who are skilled in particular areas. For example, facilitators were chosen on the basis of experience in the mental health field and in facilitating groups, as well as a commitment to reducing the prevalence of violence among youth.

Although we believe that the qualifications of the facilitator outweigh the importance of finding ethnically similar facilitators, we should note some interesting observations. In the urban area, the most qualified applicants happened to be African-American, which "matched" the target population. In the rural area, the students were more ethnically heterogeneous and it happened that there were both White and African-American facilitators. Because we have not evaluated the impact of the facilitator's ethnicity on program outcome, we cannot say for certain that having ethnically similar facilitators did or did not contribute to positive outcomes. It is also interesting to note that although there were a significant number of Hispanic students in the rural schools, none of the facilitators were Hispanic. When discussing problems in implementing the program, one facilitator noted that the Hispanic students did not want to participate in the group activities. Would having a Hispanic facilitator have changed that? We cannot say for certain, but suspect that having a qualified, skilled facilitator is more important than matching the facilitator's ethnicity to that of the students. Becoming culturally skilled is an important goal of the facilitators, which includes knowledge of and openness to different cultural groups and different world views, a willingness to explore assumptions and stereotypes that he or she might hold, recognition of the complexity of cultural issues, and acknowledgement that becoming culturally skilled is an ongoing process (Sue & Sue, 1990).

Implementation Issues

The implementation of the RIPP program represents a much more significant issue than adjusting some of the session activities or using culturally relevant language. The RIPP-6 program that we evaluated in the urban schools was implemented in 45-minute sessions once a week for 25 weeks. Process observations were conducted to ensure that the program was implemented according to the manual. Again, we have not evaluated the impact of changing the format of implementation (for example, longer or shorter sessions, more than one session a week, etc.). However, evaluations of other programs indicate that the number of sessions could impact the outcome (e.g., Aber, Jones, Brown, Chaudry, & Samples, 1998). When implementing the RIPP program, care should be taken to maintain treatment fidelity by following the lesson plans and including process observations. Having said that, we realize that there are times when the program cannot be administered exactly as planned because of various reasons, including the structure of the school, time conflicts, or the target population. This next section discusses some of the issues in program implementation and how we addressed them in the urban and rural schools. We also include a discussion of incorporating other components with RIPP, such as an after-school program or community-level intervention.

Focus

Individuals who are interested in implementing RIPP may be tempted to administer the program only to those at highest risk in at their schools. We do not, however, recommend the use of RIPP as a pull-out program. The theory upon which RIPP is based views violence as an interaction between the person, behavior, and the environment. Therefore, it would be inappropriate to target a few individual students. Given the theoretical basis of RIPP, the program is aimed at reducing specific types of violence that stem from situational or interpersonal violence. These types of violence should be distinguished from others that stem from antisocial behavior or psychopathology on the part of the perpetrator (Tolan & Guerra, 1994). RIPP therefore targets the entire population of middle school or junior high students rather than selected students. This differs from some intervention and prevention programs that target children at high-risk for antisocial behavior in order to prevent further escalation of aggression or from programs that aim to treat children who are already exhibiting chronic problems (Winett, 1998).

There have been other major problems noted with aggregating high-risk kids. In evaluating a program aimed at high-risk students, Dishion and colleagues (Dishion & Andrews, 1995; Eddy, Dishion, & Stoolmiller, 1998) noted some negative effects. Students who participated in a teen group had escalated use of tobacco and problem behaviors compared to children in the control groups. Further analyses revealed that children who had elevated levels of problem behaviors before the intervention tended to further increase their involvement in problem behaviors after being involved in the intervention. Videotaped interactions of the group sessions suggested that these children received increased attention and interest on the part of the participants and facilitator when they disclosed their involvement in problem behaviors. This attention and interest may have unintentionally reinforced their engagement in problem behaviors (Eddy et al., 1998). Others have also noted potentially harmful effects of aggregating high-risk youth (e.g., Catterall, 1987; McCord, 1992). In fact, negative effects from one program that aggregated high-risk youth continued 30 years after the program ended (Dishion, McCord, & Poulin, 1999).

Small Group Work

When we implemented the program in the rural schools, several facilitators were concerned about the small group format. They felt that some students did not adequately participate and that the groups took too much time. However, we feel very strongly about the use of group work. Cooperative learning, in which children work together in small groups to achieve a certain goal, may promote positive peer interactions, increase academic achievement, and improve self-esteem. In RIPP, the small group sessions are essential for helping children practice the skills they learn with their peers. At the same time, we acknowledge that small group work can be challenging to facilitators, especially those who don't have much experience working with such a format. There are things you can do to make small groups run more smoothly and to increase participation. The following are examples of some of the issues that were raised and how we addressed them:

1. The facilitators were concerned because students often wanted to be in groups only with their friends and would want to have the same role (e.g., leader, recorder) each time. We noted that children could be assigned to groups and group roles by the facilitator based on various factors (counting off, color of clothes). The standards for group assignment can be set early so that all children understand that they will be assigned to groups and group roles (rather than picking them).
2. Lack of group participation was noted by some facilitators, and many were confused about the "right to pass." We clarified that the "right to pass" meant that no one had to share personal information unless they wanted to, but that did not mean that they did not have to participate in group activities. For those classes where participation was a problem, we suggested that more structure be given to the children so that they would feel comfortable participating. In particular, the role-plays may be scripted in the initial sessions and then eventually allow the students to make up their own role-plays as they become more comfortable.
3. Several facilitators had classes with special education children, who often did not participate in small group activities. Some suggestions included minimizing the amount of reading necessary by reading aloud or by including more activities and providing extra attention to these students by visiting them in their other classes or telling them about the lessons beforehand (see Chapter 3 for additional suggestions for adapting RIPP for special education students).

Format

There are several issues related to the format for the RIPP program, including the length of the sessions, the timing (e.g., how many times a week), and when to have the program (e.g., during or after school). Several of these issues may depend on the scheduling characteristics of the school. For example, some schools have 45-minute classes whereas others are on a 90-minute block schedule. Moreover, there's increasing pressure for students to succeed academically and many schools don't want to allot class time to other programs. In the urban schools, for example, we had to make adjustments to the 8th grade program because the schools did not want any activities or programs to interfere with the preparation and administration of the "standards of learning" tests, which are standardized tests to measure school achievement. Because the schools were on block schedules, we rearranged the schedule so that about two sessions were combined into one. Rather than using a session-by-session format, we had the facilitators do a "running" format so that when they were completed with one session, they went directly into the next one until time ran out. Then, they picked up where they left off during the next class period. We thought that this might work because several of the sessions in the 8th grade programs had overlapping themes. For example, sessions 7 through 10 all revolve around "envisioning the future." However, the facilitators had trouble completing all of the workshops, and some components had to be dropped. We are evaluating the effects of the 8th grade program and cannot speculate on how the changes might have affected the outcome.

Another consideration is how many times a week to implement the RIPP program. In the rural schools, one of the facilitators ended up implementing the 25 sessions of the 6th grade program on a daily schedule. We were concerned about this implementation because we felt that the process of developing school norms and learning the skills taught in RIPP takes time. Bodine and Crawford (1998) noted that individuals pass through the following series of stages when learning problem-solving and conflict resolution skills: (1) having no knowledge of what skills are needed (unconsciously unskilled); (2) recognizing the need for certain skills (consciously unskilled); (3) learning to perform the skills in a rote, rehearsed manner (consciously skilled), and finally (4) being able to generalize and perform skills automatically in a variety of settings (unconsciously skilled). These stages are characterized as circular, and continued practice and honing of skills are needed to generalize skills learned in the classroom to real life scenarios. We believe that the RIPP program should be implemented no more than twice a week to allow the participants time to practice the skills between sessions. In addition, a program such as RIPP should be implemented with students at the beginning of their first year in middle or junior high school.

A final issue is when to implement the program. As mentioned previously, some schools may be hesitant to designate class time to a program and might prefer limiting RIPP to an after-school or summer program. There are, however, several advantages of implementing the program during school hours. Schools are a primary context for social development, and therefore they can provide a natural opportunity for programs that focus on teaching nonviolent strategies for addressing conflicts. The presence of prevention facilitators and peer mediators provides opportunities to help students learn how to address conflicts as they occur and can reinforce the use of skills taught by prevention programs (e.g., Aber, Brown, Chaudry, Jones, & Samples, 1996; Meyer & Farrell, 1998). Moreover, prevention facilitators can serve as models of nonviolent conflict resolution, and programs designed to permeate daily school routines can produce shifts toward recognition and reinforcement of prosocial norms. There are also practical reasons for implementing programs in school settings. Because the vast majority of children attend school, schools provide an efficient way to reach a large number of children (Samples & Aber, 1998) that avoids issues related to identifying a location, providing transportation, and ensuring program attendance (Guerra, Tolan, & Hammond, 1994). This is not to say that an after-school or summer program that included aspects and lessons from RIPP would not be appropriate, provided they are administered in conjunction with, and not as a substitution for, the classroom based program.

Increasingly, schools are becoming more aware of the need for violence prevention programs within their schools. Additionally, there is increased national attention to violence and a call for schools to address the issues of violence. For example, President Clinton recently proposed a requirement for schools to adopt a comprehensive safety plan including effective violence prevention programs (Safe and Drug Free Schools, 1999). Therefore, it is likely that issues relating to "taking time away from" class material will be reframed to acknowledge the importance of incorporating violence prevention programs into the school curriculum.

Collaboration With Other Programs

Although we feel that school-based violence prevention programs are important, we believe that the eventual goal should be implementing RIPP along with other programs and policies aimed at reducing youth violence. Collaboration among RIPP and these other programs will help to create a comprehensive program to address the multiple factors relating to violence that exist within various social domains. The exact components included in such programs depend on the needs of the specific individuals, families, schools, and communities. For example, increased police presence and improved economic opportunities may be key in certain communities. Some schools may need to address the physical environment of the school (e.g., lighting, entrances) to increase school safety. Other components include, but are not limited to, parent and/or teacher training, juvenile justice reform, improved identification and referral of high-risk students to appropriate programs, and after-school programs created or adjusted to address youth violence.

CONCLUSION

To summarize, here's what we believe works, what doesn't work, and what might:

What Works:

- Developing an understanding of the target community through critical examination, and making adaptations to the program based on this information.
- Adjusting program components in a way consistent with RIPP's framework and objectives.
- Hiring facilitators who are committed to becoming culturally skilled.
- Using culturally relevant language.
- Using procedures that help to facilitate group work and encourage all students to participate.
- Using RIPP in collaboration with other programs and policies that promote nonviolence.

What Doesn't Work:

- Making assumptions about the community or population without consulting with the management team and other sources.
- Making adaptations to the program that are inconsistent with the framework or objectives of RIPP.
- Using profanity or language that glorifies or normalizes violence.
- Using RIPP as a pull-out program that targets only high-risk students.
- Implementing RIPP so that students are not given adequate time throughout the program to incorporate and practice the skills they learn.

What Might Work:

- Matching the ethnicity of the facilitator with that of the target population.
- Making slight adjustments in timing the implementation.

Epilogue

Although we recognize that a lot of information is covered in this book, we hope that the book's comprehensiveness will help your school develop its own RIPP program. Clearly, implementation of RIPP involves dedication and commitment from the school and community staff, as well as short- and long-range planning. Fortunately, implementing RIPP can be an uplifting process that is designed to facilitate positive experiences within your school, as well as reduce violence.

In planning for RIPP, there are a few key things to remember. Most importantly, violence is a complex problem and its prevention requires efforts at multiple levels. In addition, remember that violence does not just affect "problem kids" or "problem schools"—its tentacles reach out and touch everyone. Even if violence has not profoundly touched your students or school system, nonetheless it is important to prevent violence from happening by promoting peace and positive youth outcomes. RIPP can help you do that by teaching students productive ways to promote nonviolence. For example, the RIPP-6 program teaches students how to avoid conflict by using RAID (Resolve, Avoid, Ignore, and Diffuse) and to make responsible decisions by using SCIDDLE (Stop, Calm down, Identify the problem and your feelings about it, Decide among your options, Do it, Look back, and Evaluate). In the RIPP-7 program, students learn how to use effective conflict resolution and coping strategies, especially within friendships. RIPP-8 extends the lessons learned in RIPP-6 and RIPP-7 by promoting positive risk-taking within various contexts (school, community, family), particularly in a positive transition to high school.

It is also important to remember that for RIPP to work effectively, certain things must be in place. First, a core group of school staff should be organized to act as advocates for nonviolence. This group will examine questions related to how ready your school is for RIPP programming: Do you have "buy in" from the school administration and faculty? Does your school have the time and funding for program training and implementation? How can your school evaluate RIPP? To optimize the impact of RIPP, these questions must be addressed.

Selection of the RIPP facilitator is also crucial in building an effective violence prevention program. Remember, the facilitator needs to be a "Beacon of Nonviolence." We have found that having a qualified full-time RIPP facilitator is particularly effective in preventing or reducing student conflict; if that is not possible within your school system, it is crucial that RIPP facilitators (whether they be part-time, full-time, or share responsibilities) have adequate training in RIPP programming and peer mediation.

Remember that evaluating the impact of RIPP at your school is essential. Although the word *evaluation* can conjure up words like statistics, data, and reports, evaluation itself can be enlightening and informative. Evaluation is an important and integral part of prevention—it can help define and refine the programming and show what works and what doesn't. For the first year, you might want to ease into the evaluation by considering a "pilot" year, during which you teach the curriculum to half the students and measure the results against the comparison group. You can examine the effectiveness of the program by measuring the students' knowledge, behavior, and attitudes about violence or by using school reports such as disciplinary referrals.

When implementing and evaluating the RIPP program in your school, it is helpful to remember the goals of the program. Think of RIPP as a health-promotion program, whose purpose is to teach students skills and strategies to resolve conflict and deal with issues in a peaceful and positive way. Remember that a program like RIPP cuts across risk areas because it builds protective factors that transfer across areas. The skills learned in the RIPP program may also help youth deal with other issues in their lives, such as academics and peer pressure. RIPP, when taught effectively, can promote leadership and character development. Whether RIPP is used alone or complements other preventive interventions in your school, its impact on the students, teachers, parents, and community can be powerful. Just think of the future "Beacons of Nonviolence!"

Please share your experiences with us. Contact us at:

RIPP Project
c/o Dr. Aleta Meyer
Department of Psychology
Virginia Commonwealth University
VCU Box 842018
808 W. Franklin Street
Richmond, VA 23284-2018
Phone 1-804-828-8793
Fax 1-804-828-2237

References

Aber, J. L., Brown, J. L., Chaudry, N., Jones, S. M., & Samples, F. (1996). The evaluation of the Resolving Conflict Creatively Program: An overview. *American Journal of Preventive Medicine, 5 (Suppl 2),* 82–90.

Aber, J. L., Jones, S. M., Brown, J. L., Chaudry, N., & Samples, F. (1998). Resolving conflict creatively: Evaluating the developmental effects of a school-based violence prevention program in neighborhood and classroom context. *Development and Psychopathology, 10,* 187–213.

Addis, M., Hatgis, C., Soysa, C., Zaslavsky, I., & Bourne, L. (1999). The dialectics of manual-based treatment. *The Behavior Therapist, 22,*130–132.

American Psychological Association (1992). Ethical principles of psychologists and code of conduct. Washington, DC: American Psychological Association.

Anderman, E. M., & Kimweli, D. M. (1997). Victimization and safety in schools serving early adolescents. *Journal of Early Adolescence, 17,* 408–438.

Axelson, J. A. (1993). *Counseling and development in a multicultural society.* Pacific Grove, CA: Brooks/Cole.

Bandura, A. (1986). *Social foundations of thought and action: A social cognitive theory.* Englewood Cliffs, NJ: Prentice-Hall.

Bandura, A. (1989). Human agency in social cognitive theory. *American Psychologist, 44,* 1175–1184.

Bandura, A., & Walters, R. (1959). *Adolescent aggression.* New York: Ronald Press.

Berkowitz, L. (1994). Is something missing: Some observations prompted by the Cognitive-Neoassociationistic view of anger and emotional aggression. In L. Huesmann (Ed.), *Aggressive behavior: Current perspectives* (pp. 35–57). New York: Plenum.

Bierman, K. (1989). Improving the peer relationships of rejected children. In B. Lahey, & A. Kazdin (Eds.), *Advances in clinical child psychology* (Vol. 12, pp. 53–84). New York: Plenum Press.

Bierman, K., & Montminy, P. (1993). Developmental issues in social-skills assessment and intervention with children and adolescents. *Behavior Modification, 17,* 229–254.

Bodine, R. J., & Crawford, D. K. (1998). *The handbook of conflict resolution education: A guide to building quality programs in schools.* San Francisco, CA: Jossey-Bass.

Bryant, K. J., Windle, M., & West, S. G. (Eds.) (1997). *The science of prevention: Methodological advances from alcohol and substance abuse research.* Washington, DC: American Psychological Association.

Caplan, G. (1964). *Principles of preventive psychiatry.* New York: Basic Books.

Carlo, G., Fabes, R., Laible, D., & Kupanoff, K. (1999). Early adolescence and prosocial/moral behavior II: The role of social and contextual influences. *Journal of Early Adolescence, 19,* 133–147.

Cartledge, G., & Cochran, L. (1993). Developing cooperative learning behaviors in students with behavior disorders. *Preventing School Failure, 37,* 5–10.

Catalano, R. F., Berglund, M. L., Ryan, J. A., Lonczak, H. C., & Hawkins, J. D. (1998). *Positive youth development in the United States: Research findings on evaluations of positive youth programs.* (Manuscript submitted for publication).

Catterall, J. S. (1987). An intensive group counseling dropout prevention intervention: Some cautions on isolating at-risk adolescents within high schools. *American Education Research Journal, 24,* 521–540.

Chen, H. (1990). *Theory-driven evaluations.* Newbury Park, CA: Sage.

Clark, R., Anderson, N. B., Clark, V. R., & Williams, D. R. (1999). Racism as a stressor for African-Americans: A biopsychosocial model. *American Psychologist, 54,* 805–816.

Coatsworth, J., Szapocznki, J., Kurtines, W., & Santisban, D. (1997). Culturally competent psychosocial interventions with antisocial problem behavior in Hispanic youth. In D. Stoff, J. Breiling, & J. Maser (Eds.), *Handbook of antisocial problem behavior* (pp. 395–403). New York: Wiley.

Conger, R. D., & Elder, G. H. (1994). *Families in troubled times: Adapting to change in rural America.* Hillsdale, NJ: Aldine.

Cook, T., Anson, A., & Walchli, S. (1993). From causal description to causal explanation: Improving three exemplary evaluations of adolescent health programs. In S. Millstein, A. Peterson, & E. Nightingale (Eds.), *Promoting the health of adolescents* (pp. 339–374). New York: Oxford University Press.

Cox, G. (1986). *The ways of peace.* New York: Paulist Press.

Crick, N. R. (1997). Engagement in gender normative versus nonnormative forms of aggression: Links to social-psychological adjustment. *Developmental Psychology, 33,* 610–617.

Crick, N. R., Bigbee, M. A., & Howes, C. (1996). Gender differences in children's normative beliefs about aggression: How do I hurt thee? Let me count the ways. *Child Development, 67,* 1003–1014.

Crick, N., & Dodge, K. (1994). A review and reformulation of social information-processing mechanisms in children's social adjustment. *Psychological Bulletin, 115,* 74–101.

Crick, N. R., & Grotpeter, J. K. (1995). Relational aggression, gender, and social-psychological adjustment. *Child Development, 66,* 710–722.

Crockett, L., & Petersen, A. (1993). Adolescent development: Health risks and opportunities for health promotion. In S. Millstein, A. Peterson, & E. Nightingale (Eds.), *Promoting the health of adolescents* (pp. 13–37). New York: Oxford University Press.

Crum, T. (1987). *The magic of conflict.* New York: Simon & Schuster.

Dahlberg, L. L., Toal, S. B., & Behrens, C. B. (1998). *The measurement of violence-related attitudes, beliefs, knowledge, and behavior among youth: A compendium of instruments.* Atlanta, GA: National Center for Injury Prevention and Control, National Centers for Disease Control and Prevention.

Dishion, T. J., & Andrews, D. (1995). Preventing escalation of problem behaviors with high-risk young adolescents: Immediate and 1-year outcomes. *Journal of Consulting and Clinical Psychology, 63,* 538–548.

Dishion, T. J., McCord, J., & Poulin, F. (1999). When interventions harm: Peer groups and problem behavior. *American Psychologist, 54,* 755–764.

Dishion, T. J., Patterson, G. R., & Griesler, P. C. (1994). Peer adaptations in the development of antisocial behavior: A confluence model. In L. R. Huesmann (Ed.), *Aggressive behavior: Current perspectives* (pp. 61–95). New York: Plenum.

Dodge, K. (1986). A social information processing model of social competence in children. In M.

Perlmutter (Ed.), *The Minnesota Symposium on Child Psychology* (Vol. 18, pp. 77–125). Hillsdale, NJ: Erlbaum.

Dodge, K. (1991). *On the empirical basis for preventive intervention.* Presented at the April 1991 biennial meeting of the Society for Research in Child Development, Seattle, WA.

Dusenbury, L., Falco, M., Lake, A., Brannigan, R., & Bosworth, K. (1997). Nine critical elements of promising violence prevention programs. *Journal of School Health, 67,* 409–414.

Earls, F., Cairns, R. B., & Mercy, J. A. (1993). The control of violence and the promotion of nonviolence in adolescents. In S.G. Millstein & A. C. Peterson (Eds.), *Promoting the health of adolescents: New directions for the twenty-first century* (pp. 285–304). New York: Oxford University Press.

Eddy, J. M., Dishion, T. J., & Stoolmiller, M. (1998). The analysis of intervention change in children and families: Methodological and conceptual issues embedded in intervention studies. *Journal of Abnormal Child Psychology, 26,* 53–69.

Elliott, D. S., Hamburg, B. A., & Williams, K. R. (1998). Violence in American schools: An overview. In D. S. Elliott, B. A. Hamburg, & K. R. Williams (Eds.), *Violence in American schools: A new perspective.* New York: Cambridge University Press.

Elliott, D. S., & Tolan, P. H. (1999). Youth violence prevention, intervention, and social policy: An overview. In D. J. Flannery. & C. R. Huff (Eds.), *Youth violence prevention, intervention, and social policy* (pp. 3–46). Washington, DC: American Psychiatric Press.

Eron, L. D., Gentry, J. H., &. Schlegel, P. (Eds.) (1994). *Reason to hope: A psychosocial perspective on violence and youth.* Washington, DC: American Psychological Association.

Fagan, J. (1999). Youth gangs, drugs, and socioeconomic isolation. In D. J. Flannery & C. R. Huff (Eds.), *Youth violence: Prevention, intervention, and social policy* (pp. 145–170). Washington, DC: American Psychiatric Press.

Fagan, J., & Wilkinson, D. L. (1998). Social contexts and functions of adolescent violence. In D. S. Elliott, B. A. Hamburg, & K. R. Williams (Eds.), *Violence in American schools: A new perspective.* New York: Cambridge University Press.

Farrell, A. D., Ampy, L. A., & Meyer, A. L. (1998). Identification and assessment of problematic interpersonal situations for urban adolescents. *Journal of Clinical Child Psychology, 27,* 292–305.

Farrell, A. D., Danish, S. J., & Howard, C. W. (1991). Evaluation of data screening methods in surveys of adolescents' drug use. *Psychological Assessment, 3,* 295–298.

Farrell, A. D., Howard, C. W., Danish, S. J., Smith, A. F., Mash, J. M., & Stovall, K. L. (1992). Athletes coaching teens for substance abuse prevention: Alcohol and other drug use and risk factors in urban middle school students. In C. E. Marcus & J. Swisher (Eds.) OSAP Prevention Monograph No. 12. Working with youth in high risk environments: Experiences in prevention (pp. 13–30) (DHHS Publication No. ADM 92-1815). Washington DC: U.S. Government Printing Office.

Farrell, A. D., Kung, E. M., White, K. S., & Valois, R. F. (in press). The structure of self-reported aggression, drug use, and delinquent behaviors during early adolescence. *Journal of Clinical Child Psychology.*

Farrell, A. D., & Meyer, A. L. (1997). The effectiveness of a school-based curriculum for reducing violence among sixth grade students. *American Journal of Public Health, 87,* 979–984.

Farrell, A. D., Meyer, A. L., & Dahlberg, L. (1996). Richmond Youth Against Violence: A school-based program for urban adolescents. *American Journal of Preventive Medicine, 12,* (suppl.) 13–21.

Farrell, A. D., Meyer, A. L., Kung, E. M., & Sullivan, T. N. (1999). *Development and evaluation of school-based violence prevention programs.* Manuscript submitted for publication

Farrell, A. D., Meyer, A. L., Sullivan, T. N., & Kung, E. M. (in preparation). *Evaluation of RIPP-7.*

Farrell, A. D., & Meyer, A. L., & White, K. S. (1999). *Evaluation of Responding in Peaceful and*

Positive Ways (RIPP): A school-based prevention program for reducing violence among Urban adolescents. (Manuscript submitted for publication.)

Fetterman, D. (1996). Empowerment evaluation: An introduction to theory and practice. In D. Fetterman, S. Kaftarian, & A. Wandersman (Eds.), *Empowerment evaluation: Knowledge and tools for self-assessment and accountability* (pp. 3–39). Thousand Oaks, CA: Sage.

Fitzpatrick, K. M., & Boldizar, J. P. (1993). The prevalence and consequences of exposure to violence among African-American youth. *Journal of the American Academy of Child and Adolescent Psychiatry, 32,* 424–430.

Friedlander, B. (1993). Community violence, children's development, and mass media: In pursuit of new insights, new goals, and new strategies. *Psychiatry, 56,* 66–81.

Galland, C. (1980). *Women in the Wilderness.* New York: Harper and Row.

Garbarino, J. (1982). *Children and families in the social environment.* New York: Pergamon.

Graham, S., Hudley, C., & Williams, E. (1992). Attributional and emotional determinants of aggression among African-American and Latino young adolescents. *Developmental Psychology, 20,* 619–627.

Guerra, N. G., Tolan, P. H., & Hammond, W. R. (1994). Prevention and treatment of adolescent violence. In L. D. Eron, J. H. Gentry, & P. Schlegel (Eds.), *Reason to hope: A psychosocial perspective on violence and youth.* Washington, DC: American Psychological Association.

Hamburg, M. A. (1998). Youth violence is a public health concern. In D. S. Elliot, B. A. Hamburg, & K. R. Williams (Eds.), *Violence in American schools: A new perspective* (pp. 31–54). New York: Cambridge University Press.

Hawkins, D. F., Crosby, A. E., & Hammett, M. (1994). Homicide, suicide, and assaultive violence: The impact of intentional injury on the health of African-Americans. In I. L. Livingston (Ed.), *Handbook of Black American health: The mosaic of conditions, issues, policies, and prospects* (pp. 169–189). Westport, CT: Greenwood Press.

Hawkins, J. D., Farrington, D. P., & Catalano, R. F. (1998). Reducing violence through the schools. In D. S. Elliot, B. A. Hamburg, & K. R. Williams (Eds.), *Violence in American schools: A new perspective* (pp. 188–216). New York: Cambridge University Press.

Hill, H., Soriano, F., Chen, A., & LaFromboise, T. (1994). Sociocultural factors in the etiology and prevention of violence among ethnic minority youth. In L. D. Eron, J. H. Gentry, & P. Schlegel (Eds.), *Reason to hope: A psychosocial perspective on violence and youth.* Washington, DC: American Psychological Association.

Howard, K. A., Flora, J., & Griffin, M. (1999). Violence prevention in schools: State of the science and implications for future research. *Applied and Preventative Psychology, 8,* 197–210.

Huesmann, L. (1988). An information processing model for the development of aggression. *Aggressive Behavior, 14,* 13–24.

Huesmann, L., & Miller, L. (1994). Long-term effects of repeated exposure to media violence in childhood. In L. Huessmann (Ed.), *Aggressive behavior: Current perspectives* (pp. 152–186). New York: Plenum.

Human, J., & Wassem, C. (1991). Rural mental health in America. *American Psychologist, 46,* 232–239.

Johnston, L. D. (1985). Techniques for reducing measurement error in surveys of drug use. In L. N. Robins (Ed.), *Studying drug abuse* (pp. 117–136). New Brunswick, NJ: Rutgers University Press.

Kazdin, A. E. (1998). *Research design in clinical psychology,* 3rd ed. New York: Macmillan.

Kellam, S. G. (1990). Developmental epidemiological framework for family research on depression and aggression. In G. R. Patterson (Ed.), *Depression and aggression in family interaction* (pp. 11–48). Hillsdale, NJ: Erlbaum.

Kruttschnitt, C. (1995). Violence by and against women: A comparative and cross-national analysis. In R.B. Ruback & N. A. Weiner (Eds.), *Interpersonal violent behaviors: Social and cultural aspects.* New York: Springer.

Lagerspetz, K. M., Bjorkqvist, K., & Paltonen, T. (1988). Is indirect aggression typical of females? Gender differences in aggressiveness in 11- to 12-year-old children. *Aggressive Behavior, 14,* 403–414.

Laub, J. H., & Lauritsen, J. L. (1998). The interdependence of school violence with neighborhood and family conditions. In D. S. Elliot, B. A. Hamburg, & K. R. Williams (Eds.), *Violence in American schools: A new perspective* (pp. 127–158). New York: Cambridge University Press.

Lewin, K. (1946). Action research and minority problems. *Journal of Social Issues, 2,* 34–46.

Lochman, J., & Wayland, K. (1994). Aggression, social acceptance, and race as predictors of negative adolescent outcomes. *Journal of the American Academy of Child and Adolescent Psychiatry, 33,* 1026–1035.

Loeber, R., & Stouthamer-Loeber, M. (1998). Juvenile aggression at home and at school. In D. S. Elliot, B. A. Hamburg, & K. R. Williams (Eds.), *Violence in American schools: A new perspective* (pp. 94–126). New York: Cambridge University Press.

Lowry, R., Sleet, D., Duncan, M., Powell, K., & Kolbe, L. (1995). Adolescents at risk for violence. *Educational Psychology Review, 7,* 7–39.

McCord, J. (1992). The Cambridge-Somerville Study: A pioneering longitudinal experimental study of delinquency prevention. In J. McCord & R. E. Tremblay (Eds.), *Preventing antisocial behavior: Interventions from birth through adolescence* (pp. 196–206). New York: Guilford.

McGoldrick, M., Pearce, J., & Giordano, J. (Eds.) (1982). *Ethnicity and family therapy.* New York: Guilford.

Mercy, J. A., & Potter, L. B. (1996). Combining analysis and action to solve the problem of youth violence. *American Journal of Preventive Medicine, 12* (suppl.) 1–2.

Meyer, A. L., & Farrell, A. D. (1998). Social skills training to promote resilience and reduce violence in African-American Middle School Students. *Education and Treatment of Children, 21 (4),* 461–488.

Meyer, A., & Northup, W. (1997). What is violence prevention, anyway? *Educational Leadership, May* (3), 1–33.

Meyer, A. L., & Northup, W. B. (1998). *Responding in Peaceful and Positive Ways (RIPP): A violence prevention curriculum for the sixth grade.* Richmond, VA: Virginia Commonwealth University.

Meyer, A. L., Northup, W. B., & Plybon, L. (1998). *Responding in Peaceful and Positive Ways (RIPP): A violence prevention curriculum for the seventh grade.* Richmond, VA: Virginia Commonwealth University.

Meyer, A. L., & Plybon, L. (1999). *Responding in Peaceful and Positive Ways (RIPP): A violence prevention curriculum for the eighth grade.* Richmond, VA: Virginia Commonwealth University.

Oetting, E. R., & Beauvais F. (1990). Adolescent drug use: Findings of national and local surveys. *Journal of Consulting and Clinical Psychology, 58,* 385–394.

Office for Protection from Research Risks (1991). Protection of human subjects: Title 45 Code of Federal Regulations Part 46. Washington DC: U.S. Government Printing Office.

Oliver, W. (1989). Sexual conquest and patterns of Black-on-Black violence: A structural-cultural perspective. *Violence and Victims, 4,* 257–271.

Olweaus, D. (1978). *Aggression in the schools.* New York: Wiley.

Padilla, F. (1992). *The gang as American enterprise.* New Brunswick, NJ: Rutgers University Press.

Patterson, G. (1986). Performance models for antisocial boys. *American Psychologist, 41,* 432–444.

Perry, C., & Jessor, R. (1985). The concept of health promotion and the prevention of adolescent drug abuse. *Health Education Quarterly, 12,* 169–184.

Prothrow-Stith, D. (1987). *Violence prevention curriculum for adolescents.* Newton, MA: Education Development Center.

Reiss, A. J., & Roth, J.(1993). *Understanding and preventing violence.* Washington, DC: National Academy Press.

Remboldt, C. (1998). Making violence unacceptable. *Educational Leadership, 56* (1), 32–38.

Rossi, P. H., & Freeman, H. E. (1993). *Evaluation: A systematic approach,* 5th ed.. Newbury Park, CA: Sage.

Safe and Drug Free Schools (1999). New initiatives announced at the White House conference on school safety. [on-line], Availability: http://www.ed.gov/offices/OESE/SDFS/initiati.html

Samples, F., & Aber, L. (1998). Evaluations of school-based violence prevention programs. In D. S. Elliot, B. A. Hamburg, & K. R. Williams (Eds.), *Violence in American schools: A new perspective* (pp. 217–252). New York: Cambridge University Press.

Sampson, R. J. (1993). The community context of violent crime. In W. J. Wilson (Ed.), *Sociology and the public agency* (pp. 259–286). Newbury Park, CA: Sage.

Shadish, W. R., Newman, D. L., Scheirer, M. A., & Wye, C. (Eds.) (1995). Guiding principles for evaluators. *New Directions for Program Evaluation, 66*(Summer).

Shaw, C., & McKay, H.(1969). Juvenile delinquency and urban areas. Chicago: University of Chicago Press.

Smith, T. (1996). *Raccoon circles.* Cazenovia, WI: Raccoon Institute.

Steinberg, L., Dornbusch, S., & Brown, B. (1992). Ethnic differences in adolescent achievement: An ecological perspective. *American Psychologist, 47,* 723–729.

Sue, D. W., & Sue, D. (1990). *Counseling the culturally different.* New York: Wiley.

Tolan, P., & Guerra, N. (1994). *What works in reducing adolescent violence: An empirical review of the field.* Boulder, CO: The Center for the Study and Prevention of Violence.

Tomada, G., & Schneider, B.H. (1997). Relational aggression, gender, and peer acceptance: Invariance across culture, stability over time, and concordance among informants. *Developmental Psychology, 33,* 601–609.

Valois, R., Tidwell, R., & Farrell, A. D. (1999). *Year 1 Pilot Test of RIPP in Florida.* Unpublished report.

VanSlyck, M., Stern, M., & Zak-Place, J. (1996). Promoting optimal adolescent development through conflict resolution education, training, and practice: An innovative approach for counseling psychologists. *The Counseling Psychologist, 24,* 433–461.

Warren, R. B., & Warren D. I. (1977). *The neighborhood organizer's handbook.* Notre Dame, IN: Notre Dame Press.

Weiner, B., Graham, S., & Chandler, C. (1982). Pity, anger, and guilt: An attributional analysis. *Personality and Social Psychology Bulletin, 8,* 226–232.

Wilson, W.O. (1987). *The truly disadvantaged: The innercity, underclass, and public policy.* Chicago: University of Chicago Press.

Winett, R. A. (1998). Prevention: A proactive developmental-ecological perspective. In T. H. Ollendick & M. Hersen (Eds.), *Handbook of child psychopathology* (3rd ed., pp. 637–671). New York: Plenum.

Wong, B. Y., Harris, K., & Graham, S. (1991). Academic applications of cognitive-behavioral programs with learning disabled students. In P. Kendall (Ed.), *Child and adolescent therapy: Cognitive-behavioral procedures.* New York: Guilford.

Worthington, E. L., Jr. (1998). The Pyramid model of forgiveness: Some interdisciplinary speculations about unforgiveness and the promotion of forgiveness. In Everett L. Worthington, Jr. (Ed.), *Dimensions of forgiveness: Psychological research and theological perspectives* (pp.107–138). Philadelphia: The Templeton Foundation Press.

Yung, B. R., & Hammond, W. R. (1998). Breaking the cycle: A culturally sensitive violence prevention program for African-American children and adolescents. In Lutzker (Ed.), *Handbook of child abuse research and treatment* (pp. 319–340). New York: Plenum.

Zillman, (1979). *Hostility and aggression.* Hillsdale, NJ: Erlbaum.

Index